Botulinum Neurotoxin

Botulinum Neurotoxin
A Guide to Motor Point Injections

Chong Tae Kim

Division of Rehabilitation Medicine
The Children's Hospital of Philadelphia
Professor
Perelman School of Medicine at the University of Pennsylvania

ELSEVIER

Publisher: Cathleen Sether
Acquisitions Editor: Humayra Khan
Editorial Project Manager: Sam W. Young
Project Manager: Niranjan Bhaskaran
Cover designer: Alan Studholme

3251 Riverport Lane
St. Louis, Missouri 63043

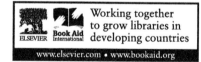

Working together to grow libraries in developing countries

www.elsevier.com • www.bookaid.org

Contents

SECTION 1 Motor points of muscles

SECTION 2 Motor points injections for deformities

Preface

Botulinum neurotoxin injection is one of the most common therapeutic options for spasticity management. Its greatest advantage overcoming disadvantages (painful, toxic, expensive) is its ability to decrease spasticity selectively. To maximize the advantage and efficiency of the injection, needless to say, it is crucial to inject the toxin into the motor points of the selected muscles. How can clinicians localize the motor points of the muscles with ease? Several reports have suggested motor points with illustration of musculoskeletal anatomy based on cadaver measurements. But these locations are not easy to be identified from the body surface. In fact, there is also some discrepancy between human body and cadaver. Some clinicians suggest most of the motor points are located at the middle part of muscle belly, but unfortunately, it is absolutely not true.

Ultrasound helps to identify the location of the muscles, but not motor points. In order to localize motor points, I would like to suggest using an electrical stimulator with mild current (less than 3 mA). In this book, I have tried to provide as many motor points as possible of almost all skeletal muscles. The most distinguished feature of this book is information on how to localize motor points of the muscles by applying surface anatomy. This is not a surface anatomy book, but a guide book for botulinum neurotoxin injection. So, brief anatomy and function are described to understand the motor point injection. In addition to the anatomy and function, some important practical tips (injection notes) are also described.

This book is composed of two parts and an appendix. Motor points of each individual muscles are illustrated in the first part. In the second part, target muscles for common deformities that result from spasticity or dystonia are discussed. Of course, no motor points localization is needed for botulinum toxin injection to the salivary and sweat glands, but the injections for drooling and sweating are described additionally in the appendix.

The author has tried to include as many muscles and deformities as possible; however, it was difficult to include all because of lack of references and the author's personal experience. I hope someday they will be included in the next edition.

I hope this book will help clinicians to improve their practice quality in botulinum toxin injection. This is the first edition of botulinum neurotoxin injection guide that applies superficial anatomy, which means it needs to be updated and revised. I really more than welcome readers' feedback, critics, and suggestions to make this book better.

Chong Tae Kim, MD, PhD

Motor points of muscles

CHAPTER

Head, face, and neck

1

1.1 Temporalis

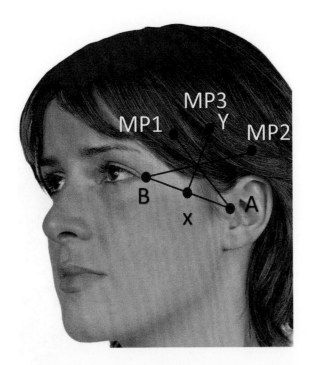

From Logan BM, Reynolds PA, Rice S, Hutchings R. McMinn's Color Atlas of Head and Neck Anatomy. 5th ed.
Elsevier; 2017: p.132.

- **Surface anatomy**: Superficial, wide, and thin muscle. Easily palpable with teeth clenching.
- **Origin**: Temporal fossa of the parietal bone.
- **Insertion**: Wide spread to the parietal, frontal, maxilla, and mandibular bone.
- **Function**: Mastication by elevation and retraction of the mandible.

Botulinum Neurotoxin. https://doi.org/10.1016/B978-0-323-69715-6.00004-1
Copyright © 2022 Elsevier Inc. All rights reserved.

- **Motor point (MP)**[1]: Three MPs. Draw a line (AB) from the tragus (A) to the lateral cantus (B), then move the line AB (A is the center) upward about 30 degrees (MP1). Move the line AB (now B is the center) upward about 30 degrees (MP2). Draw a vertical line (XY) upward (XY = AB length) from the midpoint of the AB (MP3). MP3 is relatively diffuclt to be identified than MP1 and MP2.
- **Injection tip**: The muscle is thin. If needle hits the skull, then pull the needle back. Anterior part of the muscle (MP1) is the strongest and thickest part of the muscle (because the muscle fibers run vertically), and the posterior part of the muscle (MP2) is weakest part for mastication but important function for side to side jaw movement with lateral pterygoid muscle.[2] All MPs are located in the most prominent portion of the muscle when teeth are clenched.

1.2 Masseter

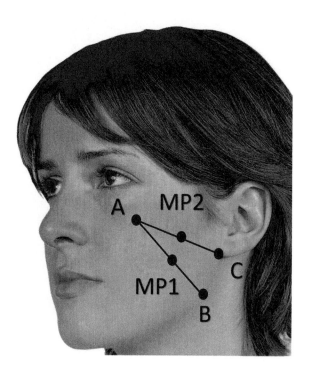

From Logan BM, Reynolds PA, Rice S, Hutchings R. McMinn's Color Atlas of Head and Neck Anatomy. 5th ed. Elsevier; 2017: p.132.

- **Surface anatomy**: Superficial muscle. Easily palpable with teeth clenching.
- **Origin**: Zygomatic process and arch of the maxilla.
- **Insertion**: Angle and ramus of the mandible.
- **Function**: Mastication by elevation and protrusion of the mandible.

- **Motor point (MP)**: The first MP (MP1) is midpoint between the maxillary process of the zygomatic bone (A) and mandibular angle (B). The second MP (MP2) is the midpoint between the zygomatic bone (A) and the distal end of ear lobule (C).
- **Injection tip**: For MP1, using thumb and the middle finger, localize the point A and B. Then place the index finger in the midpoint of the line AB. The index finger points the MP1. To avoid puncturing oral cavity, insert injection needle slowly from superficial to deep. For MP2, using thumb and the middle finger, localize the point A and C. Then place the index finger in the midpoint of the line AC. The index finger points the MP2.

1.3 Medial pterygoid

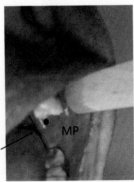

Pterygomandibular raphe   MP

- **Surface anatomy**: Very difficult to palpable extraorally.
- **Origin**: The medial side of the lateral pterygoid plate (behind of upper last molar).
- **Insertion**: Internal surface of the ramus and angle of the mandible.
- **Function**: Close the jaw with elevation of the mandible.
- **Motor point (MP)**: It is very difficult to be localized extraorally. Transoral approach is recommended. The MP in the picture shows the needle entry point to the left medial pterygoid muscle.
- **Injection tip**: At neck hyperextension and mouth opening (the most important part of the approach), localize the pterygomandibular raphe (soft tissue band connecting mandible and maxilla at the end of the last lower and upper molars). Place injection needle lateral to the upper part of the raphe and push the needle posteriorly with 30 degrees upward (toward zygomatic process) slowly. With electrical stimulation, jaw is closed if the needle is in the right place.[1,3] A long injection needle and tongue depressor are needed.

1.4 Lateral pterygoid

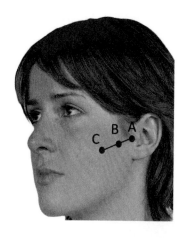

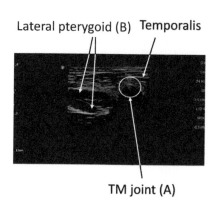

Lateral pterygoid (B) Temporalis

TM joint (A)

From Logan BM, Reynolds PA, Rice S, Hutchings R. McMinn's Color Atlas of Head and Neck Anatomy. 5th ed.
Elsevier; 2017: p.132.

- **Surface anatomy**: Located deep under the zygomatic arch and difficult to palpate.
- **Origin**: Great wing of sphenoid and pterygoid plate.
- **Insertion**: Condylar process of the mandible (just distal to the temporomandibular joint).
- **Function**: Protrusion and depression the mandible and the mandible side to side movement.
- **Motor point (MP):** Localize the temporomandibular joint (A, most prominent area) with index finger while opening and closing the mouth, and then palpate the zygomatic maxillary process with the ring finger (C). Place middle finger (B) at the midpoint of line AC. Point B is the portal of the MP of the lateral pterygoid.
- **Injection tip**: Extraoral approach is much easier than transoral approach. Ultrasound is useful to identify the TM joint and the muscle (Inset). For transoral approach, place an injection needle through the mucobuccal fold (junction of gingiva and oral mucosa) of the maxillary second molar toward to the TM joint.[1,4]

1.5 **Semispinalis capitis**

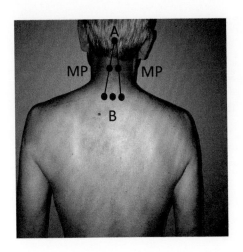
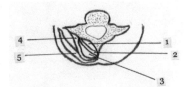

- **Surface anatomy**: Deep to the upper trapezius and splenius capitis in the posterior neck area, but superficial at the occipital area (See inset; 1. multifidus, 2. semispinalis cervicis, 3. semispinalis capitis, 4. splenius capitis, 5. splenius cervicis, 6. upper trapezius at C 6 level).
- **Origin**: Lower cervical spines and transverse processes of the upper thoracic spines.
- **Insertion**: Occipital bone medial part (just lateral to inion).
- **Function**: Extension the head.
- **Motor point (MP)**: Midpoint between inion (A) and the point just lateral to the C7 spinous process (B) and in deep (deep to the upper trapezius and splenius capitis).
- **Injection tip**: Keep head flexion as much as possible during the injection. Neck extension muscles are small and thin. They are so closely layered that it is very difficult to identify each muscle.

1.6 Semispinalis cervicis

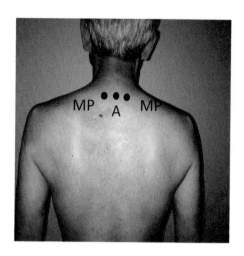
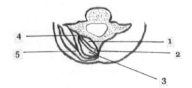

- **Surface anatomy**: The second deepest and the second most medial to the midline muscle of the posterior neck (see Inset; 1. multifidus, 2. semispinalis cervicis, 3. semispinalis capitis, 4. splenius capitis, 5. splenius cervicis, 6. upper trapezius at C 6 level).
- **Origin**: Transverse process of the upper thoracic (T1−6).
- **Insertion**: Spinous process of the upper and mid cervical spine (C2−6).
- **Function**: Extension the head and lateral flexion ipsilaterally.
- **Motor point (MP)**: 1 finger breath lateral to the C7 or T1 spinous process (A, medial to the splenius cervicis MP, see 1−8).
- **Injection tip**: MP is located in deep. Insert needle 45 degrees toward to the junction of lamina and spinous process of C7 or T1. Neck extension muscles are small and thin. They are so closely layered that it is very difficult to identify each muscle.

1.7 **Splenius capitis**

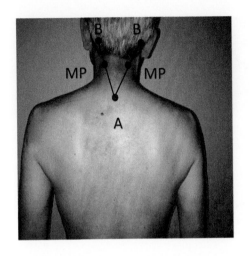 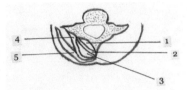

- **Surface anatomy**: Deep to upper trapezius, but superficial to semispinalis capitis in the neck (see Inset; 1. multifidus, 2. semispinalis cervicis, 3. semispinalis capitis, 4. splenius capitis, 5. splenius cervicis, 6. upper trapezius at C 6 level).
- **Origin**: Spinous processes of the lower cervical and upper thoracic spines.
- **Insertion**: To the mastoid process and the lateral occipital bone (between sternocleidomastoid and semispinalis insertions).
- **Function**: Primarily head extension, secondarily neck lateral flexion and rotation ipsilaterally.
- **Motor point (MP)**: Midpoint between C7 spinous process (A) and posterior mastoid process (B).
- **Injection tip**: Ipsilateral splenius capitis and contralateral sternocleidomastoid muscle turn head ipsilaterally (for example, right splenius capitis and left sternocleidomastoid muscle turn head to the right).

1.8 Splenius cervicis (splenius colli)

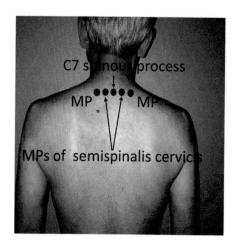

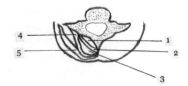

- **Surface anatomy**: Inferior and lateral to the splenius capitis at the thoracic level and deep to upper trapezius and rhomboid muscles. Narrow and long shape.
- **Origin**: Spinous processes of the third to the sixth thoracic spine.
- **Insertion**: Transverse process of the upper two or three cervical spines.
- **Function**: Extension of the cervical spine, rotation to the ipsilateral side and lateral flexion to the ipsilateral side.
- **Motor point (MP)**: Two finger breath lateral to the C7/T1 spinous process (lateral to the semispinalis cervicis MP).
- **Injection tip**: Neck extension muscles are small and thin. They are so closely layered that it is very difficult to identify each muscle. It is difficult to localize the motor point.

1.9 Longissimus capitis

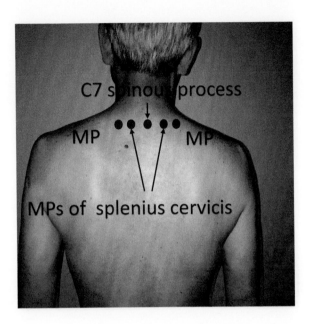

- **Surface anatomy**: Difficult to be identified because it is deep to the splenius capitis and SCM. It is medial to the longissimus cervicis.
- **Origin**: Transverse processes of the upper thoracic spines and the lower cervical spines.
- **Insertion**: Posterior mastoid process (deep to the insertions of the splenius capitis and sternocleidomastoid).
- **Function**: extension and ipsilateral rotation of the head and neck.
- **Motor point (MP)**: 3–4 finger breaths lateral to the C7/T1 spinous process (lateral to the splenius cervicis MP). Difficult to localize. Ultrasound may help identify the muscle.
- **Injection tip**: Same function as the splenius capitis but more difficult to localize the motor point.

1.10 Longissimus cervicis

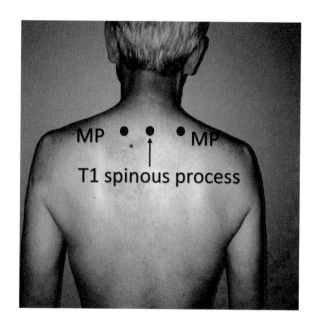

- **Surface anatomy:** Difficult to be localized. Long and thin deep muscle. Most lateral neck extensor.
- **Origin:** Transverse processes of the upper five thoracic spines.
- **Insertion:** Transverse processes of the upper cervical spines.
- **Function:** Same as longissimus capitis.
- **Motor point (MP):** 3–4 finger breaths lateral to the T1/T2 spinous process. MP is located in deep. Ultrasound may help localize the muscle.

1.11 Platysma

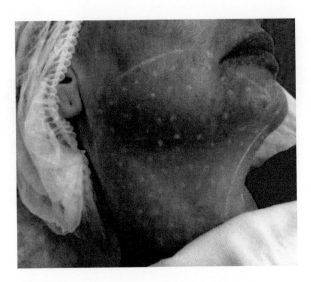

From Trindade de Almeida AR, Carruthers J. Chapter 22 - Platysma, Nefertiti Lift®, and Beyond. In: Carruthers A, Carruthers J, eds. Botulinum Toxin - Procedures in Cosmetic Dermatology Series. 4ᵗʰ ed. Elsevier; 2018

- **Surface anatomy**: Most superficial muscle covers lateral and lower face and anterior and lateral neck and very thin.
- **Origin**: Clavicle.
- **Insertion**: Lower mandible, lower lip, and cheek.
- **Function**: Depress mandible and angle of mouth.
- **Motor point (MP)**: Multiple (white dots in the picture) MPs.[5]
- **Injection tip**: The muscle can be seen and palpated when the lower lip and mandible move downward. Hold the muscle to avoid injection to the underneath muscles or organs. Inject to multiple MPs. Ultrasound helps to avoid deep injections (see Fig. A.3).

1.12 Anterior scalene (AS)

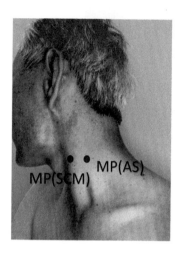

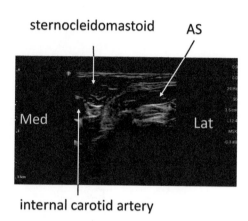

- **Surface anatomy**: Superficially located in the posterior cervical triangle lower portion (anteriorly sternocleidomastoid, posteriorly trapezius, and inferiorly clavicle), but difficult to be visualized. Palpable with shoulder elevation (levator scapulae is also palpable with shoulder elevation, but it is located in upper portion of the triangle).
- **Origin**: Cervical spine C2—C7 transverse process.
- **Insertion**: First rib.
- **Function**: Elevation the first rib and lateral flexion neck.
- **Motor point (MP)**: At supine or sitting position, MP is the midpoint of the posterior border of sternocleidomastoid .[6,7]
- **Injection tip**: Insert injection needle facing to the clavicle. Brachial plexus is located between the anterior and middle scalene muscles. If arm/finger movements is noted, the needle is close to the plexus. Ultrasound helps to identify each scalene muscle (the picture of ultrasound at mid-cervical level shows right anterior scalene, AS).

1.13 Middle scalene (MS)

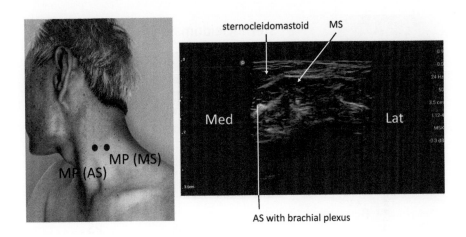

sternocleidomastoid   MS

Med   Lat

AS with brachial plexus

- **Surface anatomy**: Superficially located in the posterior cervical triangle lower portion (anteriorly sternocleidomastoid, posteriorly trapezius, and inferiorly clavicle), but difficult to be visualized. Palpable with shoulder elevation (levator scapulae is also palpable with shoulder elevation, but it is located in upper portion of the triangle).
- **Origin**: Cervical spine C3—C7 transverse process.
- **Insertion**: First rib.
- **Function**: Elevation the first rib and lateral flexion neck.
- **Motor point (MP)**: At supine or sitting position, just lateral to the anterior scalene muscle MP (see Fig. 1.12, anterior scalene muscle motor point).
- **Injection tip**: Insert injection needle facing to the clavicle (more lateral than anterior scalene muscle). Brachial plexus is located between the anterior and middle scalene muscles. If arm/finger movements is noted, the needle is close to the plexus. Ultrasound helps to identify each scalene muscle (the picture of ultrasound at mid-cervical level shows right middle scalene, MS).

1.14 Posterior scalene (PS)

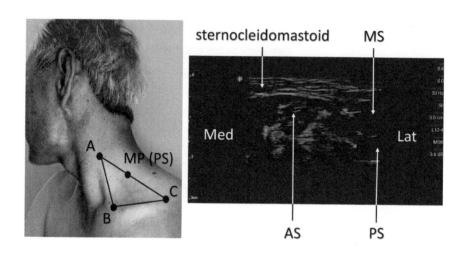

- **Surface anatomy**: Superficially located in the posterior cervical triangle lower portion (anteriorly sternocleidomastoid, posteriorly trapezius, and inferiorly clavicle), but difficult to be visualized. Palpable with shoulder elevation (levator scapulae is also palpable with shoulder elevation, but it is located in upper portion of the triangle).
- **Origin**: Cervical spine C5—C7 transverse process.
- **Insertion**: Second rib.
- **Function**: Elevation the second rib and lateral flexion neck.
- **Motor point (MP)**: At supine or sitting position, the midpoint between the anterior scalene MP (A) and the posterior angle (C) of the posterior neck triangle (ABC, B: lateral insertion point of SCM).
- **Injection tip**: Ultrasound helps to identify each scalene muscle (the picture of ultrasound at mid-cervical level shows right posterior scalene, PS).

1.15 **Sternocleidomastoid**

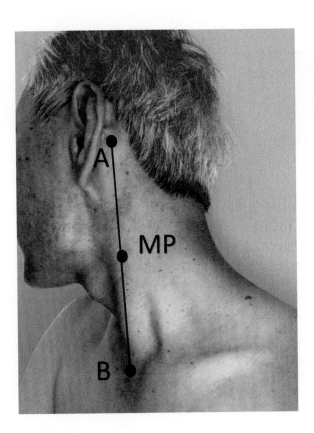

- **Surface anatomy**: Easy landmark of the neck.
- **Origin**: Manubrium and clavicle.
- **Insertion**: Mastoid process.
- **Function**: Rotation the head to the opposite side and flexion the neck.
- **Motor point (MP)**: Midpoint between mastoid (A) and manubrium (B). When inject to two sites, give each one at upper one-third and at lower one-third of the mastoid-manubrium respectively.[6,7]
- **Injection tip**: Electrical stimulation starts with low intensity. If the intensity is high, brachial plexus may be stimulated.

1.16 Longus capitis

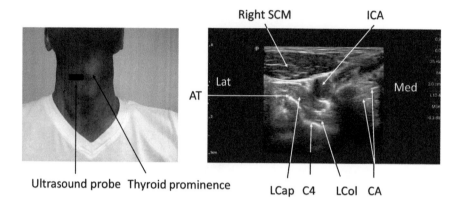

Ultrasound probe Thyroid prominence   LCap C4   LCol CA

- **Surface anatomy**: Difficult to be identified, because it is the deepest muscle of the anterior neck (behind internal carotid artery).
- **Origin**: Anterior tubercles of the transverse process of the upper cervical vertebrae (C3–6).
- **Insertion**: Occiput base
- **Function**: Flexion of the head and neck.
- **Motor point (MP)**: Unknown. Difficult to localize the muscle superficially. Ultrasound may help identify the muscle (Fig. 1.16. Right side at thyroid prominence level. AT: anterior tubercle of the C4 transverse process, C4: fourth cervical vertebra, CA: Cartilages of the thyroid and trachea, ICA: internal carotid artery, LCap: longus capitis, LCol: longus collis, SCM: sternocleidomastoid. Right internal jugular vein is compressed in this picture).
- **Injection tip**: At neck hyperextension, it is best seen by ultrasound at upper cervical vertebrae levels (localize thyroid and tracheal cartilages first at thyroid prominence level). Blind injection technique is reported[8] but not recommended personally because of risk of injury to large vessels in the neck.

1.17 **Longus collis**

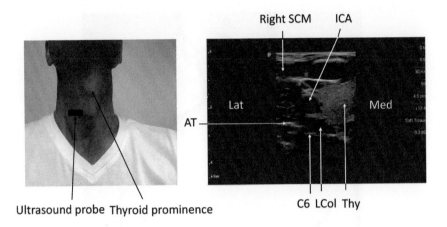

Ultrasound probe Thyroid prominence

- **Surface anatomy**: Difficult to be identified because it is the deepest muscle of the anterior neck (behind internal carotid artery and anterior to the transverse process of the cervical vertebrae).
- **Origin**: Transverse processes of the middle cervical and upper thoracic vertebrae (C5–T3).
- **Insertion**: Anterior arch of C1.
- **Function**: Flexion of the head and neck.
- **Motor point (MP)**: Unknown. Difficult to localize the muscle superficially. Ultrasound may help identify the muscle (Fig. 1.17. Left side C6 level. AT: anterior tubercle of the C6 transverse process, C6: sixth cervical vertebra, ICA: internal carotid artery, LCol: longus collis, SCM: sternocleidomastoid, Thy: thyroid gland.).
- **Injection tip**: At neck hyperextension, it is best seen by ultrasound at middle cervical vertebrae levels (localize thyroid gland and internal carotid artery first). Blind injection technique is reported[8] but not recommended personally because of risk of injury to large vessels in the neck.

1.18 Levator scapulae

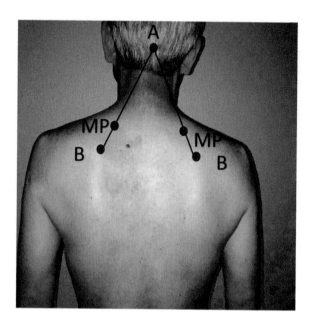

- **Surface anatomy**: Mostly covered with upper trapezius, but becomes superficial in the posterior cervical triangle upper portion (palpable with shoulder elevation, but scalene is also palpated in the lower portion). However, posterior approach is easy to localize the motor point.
- **Origin**: Transverse processes of C1−4.
- **Insertion**: Medial border of the scapula extending from superior angle to junction of spine and medial border of scapula.
- **Function**: Elevation and rotation the shoulder.
- **Motor point (MP)**: Posterior approach is easier to identify MP. At sitting, distal one-fourth between the inion (A) and supeiror angle of the scapula (B) (levator scapulae muscle is covered with upper trapezius at this point).

1.19 **Upper trapezius**

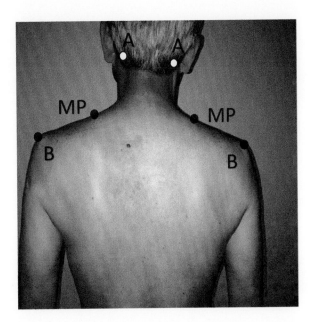

- **Surface anatomy**: Thin superficial muscle of the upper back and neck.
- **Origin**: Spinous process of C1−C7 vertebrae.
- **Insertion**: Wide insertion to the inion, occipital bone, and posterior border of the latera third of the clavicle.
- **Function**: Rotation acromion of the scapular toward the ear.
- **Motor point (MP)**: Superficially located, mid portion of the neck curve AB (from the matsoid, A to the shoulder lateral tip, B).
- **Injection tip**: The muscle is the most superficial layer. Do not push injection needle too deep.

1.20 Middle trapezius

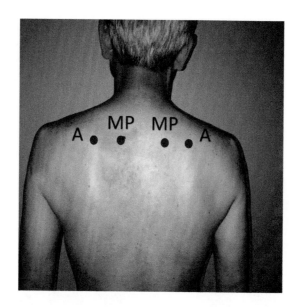

- **Surface anatomy**: Middle part of trapezius and thin superficial muscle covering supraspinatus area of scapula and rhomboid muscles.
- **Origin**: Spinous process of C7–T3 vertebrae.
- **Insertion**: Acromion and scapular spine.
- **Function**: Stabilization and retraction scapular.
- **Motor point (MP)**: Superficially located, just 1–2 finger breath medial to the point (A) where scapular spine and scapular medial border meet.
- **Injection tip**: This muscle is the most superficial layer. To avoid injecting into the rhomboid minor muscle, please keep the needle superficially.

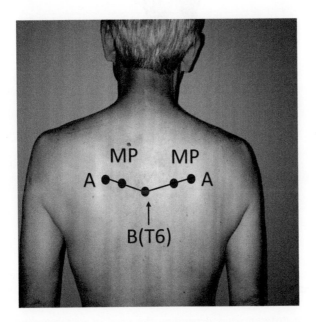

Trunk

2.1 Lower trapezius

- **Surface anatomy**: Lower part of trapezius and thin superficial muscle covering parts of scapula and rhomboid muscles.
- **Origin**: Spinous process of T4–T12 vertebrae.
- **Insertion**: Scapular spine.
- **Function**: Stabilization, retraction, and rotation scapular upward rotation (from posterior view).

Botulinum Neurotoxin. https://doi.org/10.1016/B978-0-323-69715-6.00005-3

- **Motor point (MP)**: Superficially located, lateral one-third between midpoint (A) of medial border of scapula and spinous process (B, here T6 spinous process).[9]
- **Injection tip**: This muscle is the most superficial layer. To avoid injecting into the rhomboid muscles, please keep the needle superficially.

2.2 Paraspinal muscles

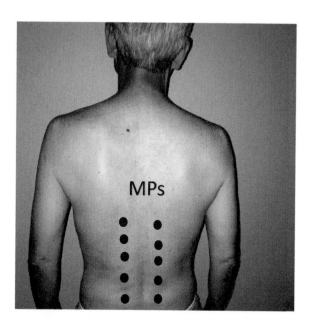

- **Surface anatomy**: Bilateral muscle groups along the spinous processes of vertebrae.
- **Origin**: From different sites depending the level of vertebrae and the depth of muscles.
- **Insertion**: To different sites depending the level of vertebrae and the depth of muscles.
- **Function**: Extension the back.
- **Motor point (MP)**: Most eminent point of each vertebral level.[10]
- **Injection tip**: Insert the needle at prone or side lying positon. For multiple level injections, keep the injection distances at 2−3 vertebral levels.

Upper arm

3.1 Pectoralis major

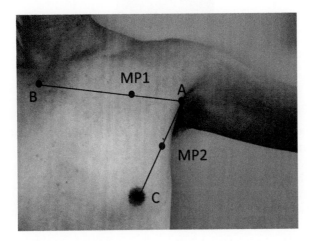

- **Surface anatomy**: Superficial and thick muscle.
- **Origin**: Wide origin area such as medial clavicle, sternum, and cartilages of all ribs.
- **Insertion**: Narrowly converge to upper humerus anteromedial site (bicipital groove).
- **Function**: Shoulder adduction and medial (internal) rotation.
- **Motor point (MP)**: MP1, lateral 1/3 point between anterior axillary fold (A) and suprasternal notch (B)[10]. MP2, mid-point between anterior axillary fold (A) and nipple (C).

Botulinum Neurotoxin. https://doi.org/10.1016/B978-0-323-69715-6.00006-5

- **Injection tip:** The MP1 is in deep (MP2 is not as deep as MP1). Pneumothorax can be prevented, as long as the needle is not deeper than 4 cm (in adult). At supine or sitting position, abduct the shoulder about 60 degrees and then grab the pectoralis muscle lateral part with one hand. It helps to estimate the needle depth. If elbow or hand movement is noticed, the needle is close to the brachial plexus.

3.2 Corachobrachialis

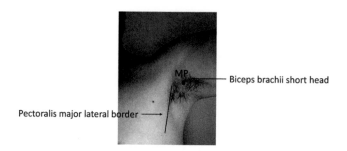

- **Surface anatomy**: Just medial and posterior to biceps brachii short head.
- **Origin**: Coracoid process of scapula.
- **Insertion**: Medial humerus.
- **Function**: shoulder adduction and flexion.
- **Motor point (MP)**: MP is just inferior to the short head of biceps brachii where the lateral border of the pectoralis major meets medial border of short head of biceps brachii.
- **Injection tip**: Needs shoulder abduction (about 90 degrees) to identify the muscle. Starting with low electric stimulation. MP is close to the axillary artery and musculocutaneous nerve. Insert needle toward the acromion to avoid the nerve stimulation (if needle is close to the nerve, significant elbow flexion is noted) and axillary artery puncture. MP is adequately stimulated, only shoulder adduction without elbow flexion can be seen.

3.3 **Latissimus dorsi**

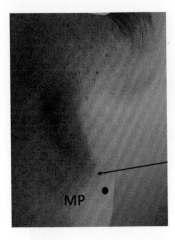

Scapular inferior angle

MP

- **Surface anatomy**: Superficial, flat, large muscle on the lateral part of back. It runs lateral to the scapula.
- **Origin**: Lower thoracic and all lumbar spine, thoracolumbar fascia, and iliac crest.
- **Insertion**: Upper humerus anteromedial site (bicipital groove).
- **Function**: Shoulder adduction, medial (internal) rotation, and extension.
- **Motor point (MP)**: Two-three finger breadths inferolateral to the inferior scapular angle[10].
- **Injection tip**: At side lying position, identify the scapular inferior angle. Two-three finger breadths inferolateral to the scapular angle. Since this is thin flat muscle, grab this area with one hand and then insert a needle slowly (45 degrees to the surface). To prevent pneumothorax, do not insert a needle through intercostal area.

3.4 Supraspinatus

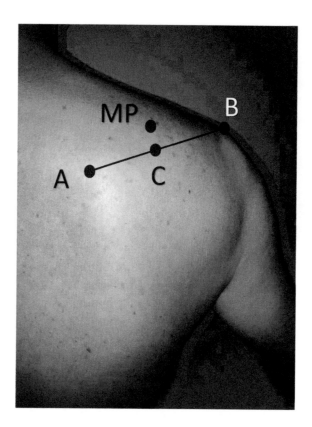

- **Surface anatomy**: Deep to upper trapezius muscle. Scapula spine separates supraspinatus and infraspinatus. Palpable with shoulder abduction only.
- **Origin**: Supraspinatus fossa of scapula.
- **Insertion**: Greater tubercle of humerus.
- **Function**: Shoulder abduction and lateral (external) rotation.
- **Motor Point (MP)**: 1–2 finger breaths superior to the midpoint (C) between the point (A) where scapular spine meets medial border of the scapula and acromion lateral tip (B).
- **Injection tip**: At sitting or side lying positon, make sure the needle passes through upper trapezius. If the needle hit the scapula, then draw the needle slowly backward.

3.5 Infraspinatus

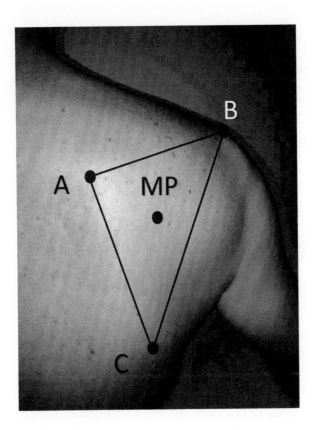

- **Surface anatomy**: Deep to mid trapezius muscle. Scapula spine separates infraspinatus and supraspinatus.
- **Origin**: Infraspinatous fossa of the scapula.
- **Insertion**: Greater tubercle of the humerus.
- **Function**: Lateral (external) rotation of the shoulder.
- **Motor point (MP)**: Center of the infraspinous fossa (center of triangle ABC, A: point where scapular spine meets medial border of scapula, B: acromion, C: inferior angle).
- **Injection tip**: At prone, sitting, or side lying position, insert the needle through the center of the infraspinous fossa. The needle has to penetrate mid-trapezius muscle. If the needle hits the bone (scapula), draw the needle backward slowly.

3.6 Subscapularis

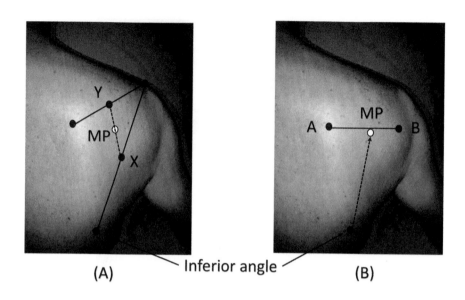

(A)   Inferior angle   (B)

- **Surface anatomy:** It is not visible or palpable.
- **Origin:** Subscapular fossa.
- **Insertion:** Lesser tubercle of humerus.
- **Function:** Shoulder internal (medial) rotation.
- **Motor point (MP):** Two (lateral and medial) approaches.
  - **(A)** <u>Lateral approach</u>: At prone position with shoulder flexion, mark a midpoint (X) between inferior scapular angle and acromion tip. From the point X, insert the needle toward a midpoint (Y) between the scapular spine medial end and acromion tip. Slowly proceed the needle until to reach the midpoint of line XY[11] (Fig. A).
  - **(B)** <u>Medial approach</u>: At prone position with shoulder internal rotation, insert the needle upward about 10 cm (in adult case) through inferior scapular angle toward the mid-part of the line AB (A, from scapular spine medial end to B, lateral border of scapular)[12] (Fig. B).
- **Injection tip:** Needs a long injection needle for both approaches. When the needle hits the bone (subscapular fossa), the needle just penetrates the muscle. In this case, slowly pull the needle back.

3.7 **Rhomboid major**

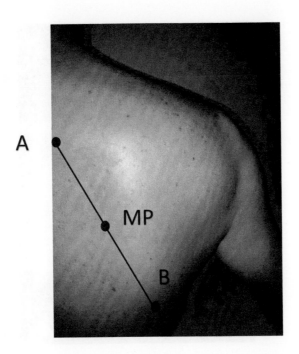

- **Surface anatomy**: Deep to the mid-trapezius.
- **Origin**: Spinous processes of upper thoracic spines.
- **Insertion**: Medial border lower part of the medial border of scapula.
- **Function**: Scapular retraction and rotation downward laterally.
- **Motor point (MP)**: Midpoint between T3 or T4 spinous process (A) and the point where ipsilateral scapular inferior angle (B).
- **Injection tip**: At prone (or side lying) position, the needle has to penetrate mid-trapezius muscle. To prevent pneumothorax, dose not insert the needle through the intercostal areas.

3.8 Rhomboid minor

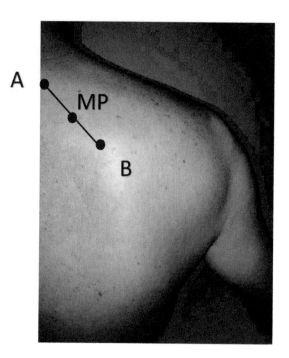

- **Surface anatomy**: Deep to the upper and mid-trapezius.
- **Origin**: Spinous processes of the lower cervical spines.
- **Insertion**: Medial border upper part of the medial border of scapula.
- **Function**: Scapular retraction and rotation downward laterally.
- **Motor point (MP)**: Midpoint between C7 or T1 spinous process (A) and the point where scapular spine meets medial border of the scapula (B).
- **Injection tip**: At prone (or side lying) position, the needle has to penetrate upper and/or mid-trapezius muscle. To prevent pneumothorax, dose not insert the needle through the intercostal areas.

3.9 **Serratus anterior**

Anterior axillary fold to iliac crest peak

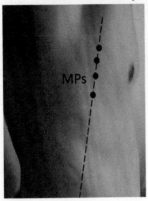

- **Surface anatomy**: Superficial between latissimus dorsi and pectoralis major. Composed of eight or nine small muscles.
- **Origin**: Lateral part of upper 8–9 ribs.
- **Insertion**: Medial border of the scapula.
- **Function**: Protraction and upward rotation of the scapula.
- **Motor point (MP)**: Each small muscles have own MP in the center of each muscle. MP is located at the point of each rib along the line from the anterior axillary fold toward the peak of the ipsilateral iliac crest.
- **Injection tip**: At side lying position, abduct the arm about 90 degrees and mark the lateral border of the pectoralis major and latissimus dorsi. This is superficial muscle. Confirm the needle hit the rib to prevent pneumothorax.

3.10 Teres major

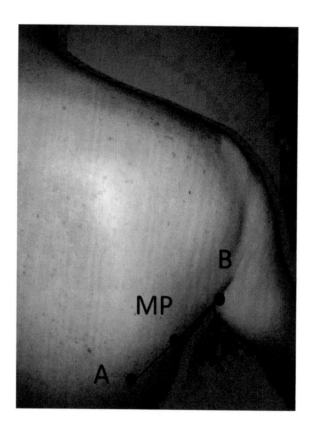

- **Surface anatomy**: Forms posterior wall of axilla and superior to latissimus dorsi.
- **Origin**: Posterior aspect of scapula angle.
- **Insertion**: Bicipital groove of the humerus.
- **Function**: Adduction and internal rotation of the shoulder.
- **Motor point (MP)**: Midpoint between scapular inferior angle (A) and starting point of the posterior axillary line (B).
- **Injection tip**: At side lying or sitting position, abduct the arm about 90 degrees.

3.11 **Teres minor**

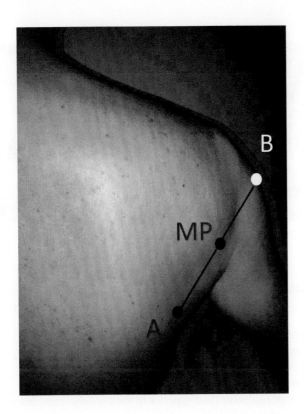

- **Surface anatomy**: It is located superior to teres major. Superficial in the triangle formed by teres major (inferiorly), scapula lateral border (laterally), and posterior deltoid muscles (superiorly).
- **Origin**: Lateral border of the scapula.
- **Insertion**: Greater tubercle of the humerus.
- **Function**: External (lateral) rotation of the shoulder.
- **Motor point (MP)**: Midpoint between distal one-third (A) of the lateral scapular borderline and shoulder lateral tip (B).
- **Injection tip**: At side lying (or prone) position, abduct about 90 degrees and then external rotate the arm. The MP is located just posterior to the deltoid posterior part.

3.12 **Deltoid**

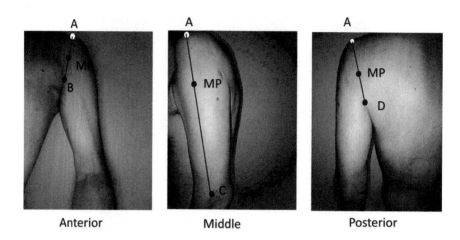

Anterior   Middle   Posterior

- **Surface anatomy**: Three parts (anterior, middle, and posterior).
- **Origin**: Lateral third of the clavicle (anterior), acromion (lateral), spine of scapula (posterior).
- **Insertion**: Deltoid tuberosity of the humerus.
- **Function**: Shoulder abduction (middle part), flexion (anterior part), and extension (posterior part).
- **Motor points (MPs)**[10]:
  1) <u>Anterior part</u>: midpoint (just superior to the cephalic vein) between acromion (A) and anterior axilla (B).
  2) <u>Middle part</u>: midpoint (very close to the bulkiest area of the muscle) between the acromion (A) and upper one-third of the lateral epicondyle (C).
  3) <u>Posterior part</u>: midpoint between the acromion (A) and posterior axilla (D).

3.13 **Biceps brachii**

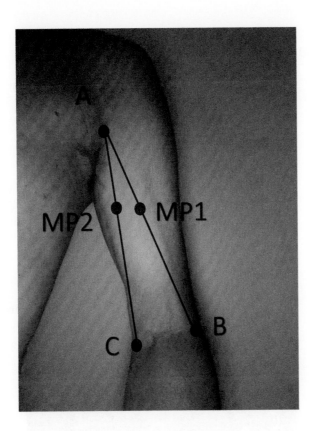

- **Surface anatomy**: Two heads (long and short head); short head is medial.
- **Origin**: Long head: coracoid process of the scapula.
  Short head: supraglenoid tubercle of the scapula.
- **Insertion**: Radial tuberosity.
- **Function**: Flexion the elbow. Supination forearm at elbow extension position.
- **Motor points (MPs)**[9,10]:
  1) Long head (**MP1**): upper one-third point between axilla (A) and lateral elbow (B).
  2) Short head (**MP2**): upper one-third point between axilla (A) and medial elbow (C).
- **Injection tip**: At side lying or sitting position, abduct the arm and supinate the forearm (biceps brachii is a major elbow flexor at forearm supinated position).

Approach from the medial side for short head and from the lateral side for long head. The motor points (for both heads) are superficial. Biceps brachii is a primary elbow flexor at forearm supination.

3.14 Triceps brachii

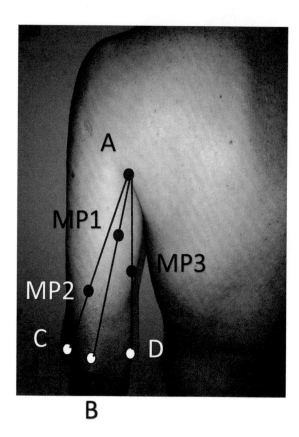

- **Surface anatomy**: From posterior view of the arm, long head lies most medially; lateral head laterally, and medial head in between.
- **Origin**: Long head: infraglenoid tubercle of scapula.
  Lateral head: above the radius sulcus of humerus.
  Medial head: below the radius sulcus of humerus.
- **Insertion**: Olecranon of ulna.

- **Function**: Extension forearm (long head extends shoulder too).
- **Motor points (MPs)**[10]:
  1) <u>Long head (**MP1**)</u>: upper one-third between axilla (A) and olecranon (B).
  2) <u>Lateral head (**MP2**)</u>: lower one-third between axilla (A) and lateral epicondyle (C).
  3) <u>Medial head (**MP3**)</u>: midpoint between axilla (A) and medial epicondyle (D).

3.15 **Brachialis**

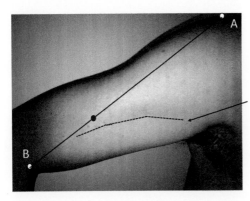

Biceps brachii

- **Surface anatomy**: Most of the muscle is deep to the biceps brachii.
- **Origin**: Distal one-third of the humerus anterior surface.
- **Insertion**: Coronoid process and tuberosity of the ulna.
- **Function**: Elbow flexion at forearm pronated position.
- **Motor point (MP)**: Distal one-third point between the acromion (A) and the lateral elbow (B).
- **Injection note**: At side lying or supine position, keep the shoulder abducted and the elbow flexed and the forearm pronated (positioning is very important). Approach from the lateral side is suggested to keep the needle away from the nerves and vessels. Insert the needle between the biceps brachii and humerus bone. Make sure the elbow flexion at forearm pronated positon with electrical stimulation (brachialis is a major elbow flexor at forearm pronated position).

Forearm

4.1 Brachioradialis

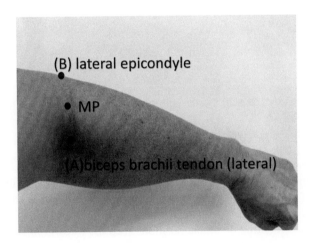

- **Surface anatomy**: Lateral border of the antecubital fossa and palpable with forearm flexion at neutral position.
- **Origin**: Lateral supracondylar ridge of the distal humerus.
- **Insertion**: Radial styloid process (distal radius).
- **Function**: Elbow flexion at forearm neutral position.
- **Motor point (MP)**: Midpoint between biceps brachii tendon (lateral side, A) and lateral epicondyle (B)[13].
- **Injection tip**: At sitting or supine position, keep the forearm in neutral position and elbow flexion 30–40 degrees (positioning is very important). MP is superficial. Make sure the elbow flexion at forearm neutral position with electrical stimulation (brachialis is a major elbow flexor at forearm neutral position).

Botulinum Neurotoxin. https://doi.org/10.1016/B978-0-323-69715-6.00008-9

4.2 Pronator teres

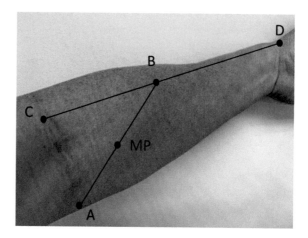

- **Surface anatomy**: Medial border of the antecubital fossa and palpable with forearm pronation.
- **Origin**: Medial supracondylar ridge of distal humerus.
- **Insertion**: Middle of the lateral surface of the radius.
- **Function**: Pronation of forearm and elbow flexion.
- **Motor point (MP)**: Midpoint between the medial epicondyle of the elbow (A) and half point of the lateral forearm (B). B is the midpoint between lateral antecubital fossa (C) and wrist lateral end (D).
- **Injection tip**: At sitting or supine position, keep the forearm in neutral position and slight elbow flexion (about 30 degrees). The muscle is superficial. If the needle is inserted deep, it may stimulate median nerve and wrist/finger flexors. Make sure the forearm pronation without finger or wrist flexion with electrical stimulation.

4.3 **Pronator quadratus**

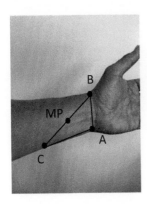

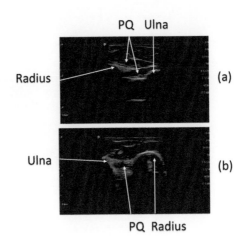

- **Surface anatomy**: It lies deep to the distal anterior of forearm and runs obliquely from ulnar to radius.
- **Origin**: Distal one-quarter of the anterior ulnar.
- **Insertion**: Distal end of the anterior radius.
- **Function**: Forearm pronation when elbow is flexed.
- **Motor point (MP)**: Draw a line of twice length of the wrist (volar side, line AB) from the wrist ulnar end (point A) upward along the ulnar side (point C) ($2 \times AB = AC$), then draw another line to the wrist radius end (point B). MP is the midpoint of the line BC.
- **Injection tip**: It is deep to the tendons of wrist-finger flexors. Make sure pronation of the forearm at elbow flexion position (pronator quadratus is a major forearm pronator at elbow flexion position). To minimize the median nerve stimulation, insert the needle through the medial side of palmaris longus tendon. Volar approach (described here) is recommended in two reasons. First, dorsal approach needs forearm pronation so it is difficult to see pronation with electrical stimulation and second, this muscle has narrower widow between the radius and ulnar at forearm pronated position (ultrasound image of the left forearm, b) than at forearm supinated (ultrasound image of the left forearm, a).

4.4 Palmaris longus

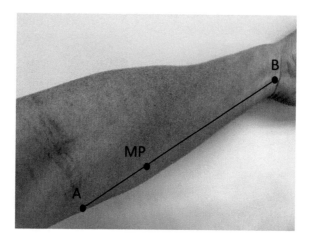

- **Surface anatomy**: Superficial and small located between flexor carpi radialis and flexor carpi ulnaris. Not always present (15% population absent). Prominent with wrist flexion.
- **Origin**: Medial supracondylar ridge of distal humerus.
- **Insertion**: Mid-wrist (palmar aponeurosis).
- **Function**: Wrist flexion.
- **Motor point**: Proximal one-third between medial epicondyle (A) and midpoint of distal wrist crease (Palmaris longus tendon insertion) (B).
- **Injection tip**: At sitting or supine position, keep the forearm in supinated position. The muscle is superficial. If Insert the needle deep, it may stimulate median nerve and/or wrist and finger flexors.

4.5 **Flexor carpi radialis**

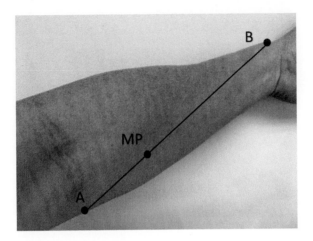

- **Surface anatomy**: Superficial and medial to the pronator teres.
- **Origin**: Medial supracondylar ridge of the distal humerus.
- **Insertion**: Second and third metacarpal bones.
- **Function**: Wrist flexion and radial deviation.
- **Motor point (MP)**: Proximal one-third point of the line between medial epicondyle (A) and wrist radial end (B).
- **Injection tip**: At sitting or supine position, keep the forearm in supinated position. The muscle is superficial. If Insert the needle deep, it may stimulate median nerve and/or finger flexors. Make sure the wrist flexion without finger flexion.

4.6 Flexor carpi ulnaris

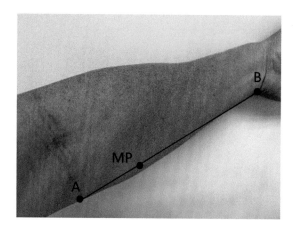

- **Surface anatomy**: Superficial and medial side of the forearm volar side.
- **Origin**: Medial supracondylar ridge of distal humerus.
- **Insertion**: Carpal bones and fifth metacarpal bone.
- **Function**: Wrist flexion and ulnar deviation.
- **Motor point (MP)**: Proximal one-third between medial epicondyle (A) and wrist joint ulnar end (B).[14]
- **Injection tip**: At sitting or supine position, keep the arm abduction and forearm supination. If the needle is inserted deeply, it may stimulate ulnar nerve and/or finger flexors.

4.7 **Flexor digitorum superficialis**

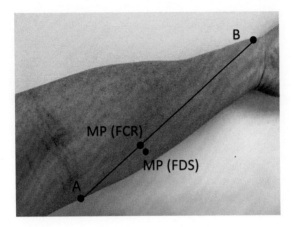

- **Surface anatomy**: Deep to the pronator teres, flexor carpi radialis and ulnaris.
- **Origin**: Medial supracondylar ridge of the distal humerus.
- **Insertion**: Middle phalanges.
- **Function**: Flexion ginger proximal interphalangeal joints.
- **Motor point (MP)**: Slight medial to MP of flexor carpi radialis (see 4–5).
- **Injection tip**: At sitting or supine position, keep the forearm in supinated position. The muscle is deep. MP is very close to the MPs of flexors carpi radialis and ulnaris. Make sure the finger PIP joint flexion without DIP joint flexion.

4.8 Flexor digitorum profundus

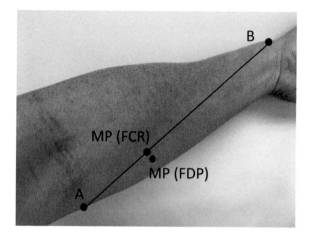

- **Surface anatomy**: Deep to the pronator teres, flexor carpi radialis and ulnaris.
- **Origin**: Proximal ulnar volar and medial side.
- **Insertion**: Distal phalanges.
- **Function**: Flexion finger distal and proximal interphalangeal joints.
- **Motor point (MP)**: Slight medial to MP of flexor carpi radialis (same location as flexor digitorum superficialis, see 4–5 and 4–7), but deeper than MP of flexor digitorum superficialis. It is very difficult to differentiate the two MPs between flexors digitorum superficialis and profundus via superficial approach.
- **Injection tip**: At sitting or supine position, keep the forearm in supinated position. The muscle is deep. Make sure prominent DIP joint flexion than PIP joint flexion.

4.9 **Flexor pollicis longus**

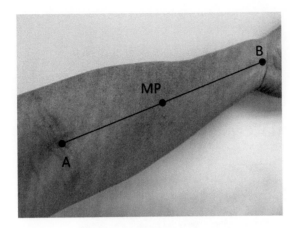

- **Surface anatomy**: Deep to the brachioradialis laterally and flexor carpi radialis medially (hard to identify this muscle superficially).
- **Origin**: Mid-radius anterior portion and interosseous membrane.
- **Insertion**: Distal phalanx of the thumb.
- **Function**: Flexion thumb interphalangeal joint.
- **Motor point (MP)**: Midpoint between biceps brachii tendon lateral side at the elbow (A) and flexor carpi radialis tendon at the wrist (B). MP is deep between brachioradialis tendon (lateral) and flexor carpi radialis tendon (medial).
- **Injection tip**: At sitting or supine position, keep the forearm in supinated position. The muscle is deep. First, confirm brachioradialis tendon laterally and flexor carpi radialis tendon medially, and then insert the needle between the two tendons, and then down to the radius. If the needle hits the radius, slowly drawback the needle. Make sure isolated thumb IP joint flexion with electrical stimulation.

4.10 Extensor carpi radialis longus

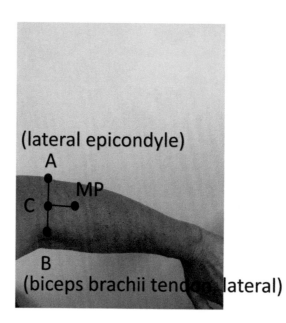

- **Surface anatomy**: At forearm pronated position, just lateral to the brachioradialis muscle.
- **Origin**: Lateral supracondylar ridge (common extensor origin site).
- **Insertion**: Second metacarpal.
- **Function**: Extension wrist to the radial side.
- **Motor point (MP)**: Mark a midpoint (C) between lateral epicondyle (A) and biceps brachii tendon insertion at the elbow (B). The MP of extensor carpi radialis longus is located at the same length of the line (AC or BC) distal to the point C (AC = BC = CMP).
- **Injection tip**: At sitting or supine position, keep the forearm in pronated position. Just distal to the brachioradialis muscle groove.

4.11 **Extensor carpi radialis brevis**

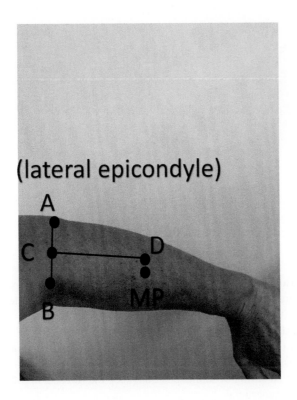

- **Surface anatomy**: At forearm pronated position, just lateral to the extensor carpi radialis longus.
- **Origin**: Lateral supracondylar ridge (common extensor origin site).
- **Insertion**: Third metacarpal.
- **Function**: Extension wrist to the radial side.
- **Motor point (MP)**: Mark a midpoint (C) between lateral epicondyle (A) and biceps brachii tendon insertion at the elbow (B). Draw a line from the point C distally to point D (CD = 2 × AB). MP of the extensor carpi radialis brevis is located slightly toward the radius.
- **Injection tip**: At sitting or supine position, keep the forearm in pronated position. The muscle is superficial.

4.12 Extensor carpi ulnaris

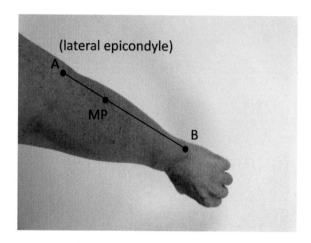

- **Surface anatomy**: At pronated position, most lateral side of proximal forearm
- **Origin**: Lateral supracondylar ridge (common extensor origin site).
- **Insertion**: Fifth metacarpal.
- **Function**: Extension wrist to the ulnar side.
- **Motor point (MP)**: Proximal one-third between lateral epicondyle (A) and ulnar styloid process (B).
- **Injection tip**: At sitting or supine position, keep the forearm in pronated position. The muscle is superficial.

4.13 Extensor digitorum communis

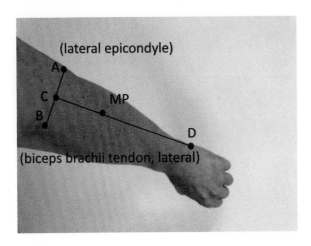

- **Surface anatomy**: Positioned in the mid portion of forearm dorsal aspect; most prominent muscle of the upper forearm (dorsal aspect) with wrist and finger extension.
- **Origin**: Lateral supracondylar ridge (common extensor origin site).
- **Insertion**: Distal phalanges from second to fifth fingers.
- **Function**: Extension wrist and fingers.
- **Motor point (MP)**: Mark a midpoint (C) between lateral epicondyle (A) and biceps brachii tendon insertion at the elbow (B). The MP of extensor digitorum communis is located at proximal one-third of the line between point C and ulnar styloid process (D). More ulnar side to the MP of extensor carpi radialis brevis (see 4–11).
- **Injection tip**: At sitting or supine position, keep the forearm in supinated position. The muscle is superficial. May see individual finger extension depending on the needle sites.

4.14 Abductor pollicis longus

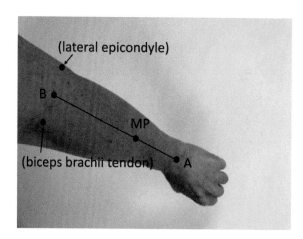

- **Surface anatomy**: Becomes superficial from the mid portion of the forearm dorsal aspect and runs obliquely to the thumb.
- **Origin**: Proximal radius and ulnar and interosseous membrane.
- **Insertion**: First metacarpal.
- **Function**: Abduction thumb and assists thumb extension.
- **Motor point (MP)**: Distal one-third (MP) of the line between midpoint (A) of wrist dorsum and mid-point (B) between biceps tendon at elbow and lateral epicondyle.
- **Injection tip**: At sitting or supine position, keep the forearm in pronated position. The muscle is superficial and proximal to the extensor pollicis brevis.

4.15 Extensor pollicis longus

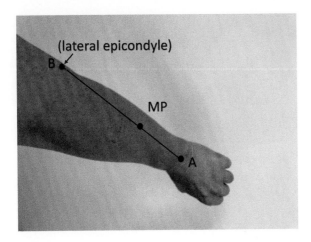

- **Surface anatomy**: Becomes superficial from the lower one-third portion of the forearm dorsal aspect and runs obliquely to the thumb.
- **Origin**: Middle ulnar and interosseous membrane.
- **Insertion**: Thumb distal phalanx.
- **Function**: Extension thumb at metacarpophalangeal and interphalangeal joints.
- **Motor point** (MP): Distal one-third (MP) of the line between midpoint (A) of wrist dorsum and lateral epicondyle (B). Slight lateral (toward ulnar) to MP of abductor pollicis longus (4.14).
- **Injection tip**: At sitting or supine position, keep the forearm in pronated and slightly elbow flexed position. The MP is deep to the extensor digitorum communis muscle.

4.16 Extensor pollicis brevis

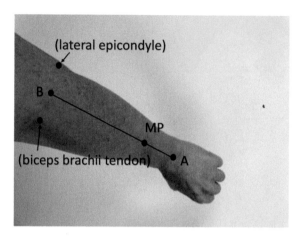

- **Surface anatomy**: Becomes superficial from the lower one-third portion of the forearm dorsal aspect and runs obliquely to the thumb.
- **Origin**: Radius and interosseous membrane.
- **Insertion**: Thumb proximal phalanx.
- **Function**: Extension thumb at metacarpophalangeal joint.
- **Motor point (MP)**: Distal one-fourth (MP) of the line between midpoint (A) of wrist dorsum and mid-point (B) between biceps tendon at elbow and lateral epicondyle (distal to MP of the abductor pollicis longus, 4–14).
- **Injection tip**: At sitting or supine position, keep the forearm in pronated and slightly flexed position. The muscle very closely lies with the abductor pollicis longus. This muscle is slightly lateral (ulnar side) and distal to the abductor pollicis longus.

4.17 **Extensor indicis**

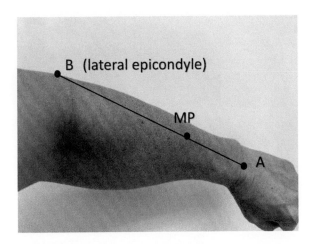

- **Surface anatomy**: Deep muscle becomes superficial only at the distal forearm (dorsal aspect).
- **Origin**: Distal ulnar and interosseous membrane.
- **Insertion**: Index finger.
- **Function**: Extension index finger.
- **Motor point (MP)**: Distal one-third (MP) of the line between midpoint (A) of wrist dorsum and lateral epicondyle (B). This is slightly ulnar side to MP of the extensor pollicis longus (see 4–15).
- **Injection tip**: At sitting or supine position, keep the forearm in pronated and slightly flexed position. MP is located in deep and close to the extensor pollicis longus MP. Make sure isolated index finger extension with electrical stimulation.

4.18 Supinator

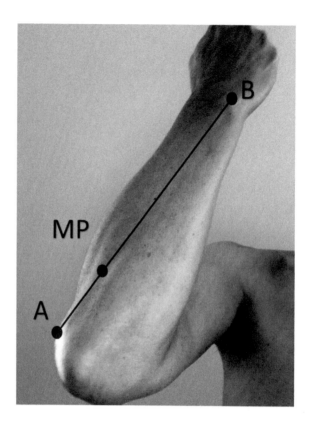

- **Surface anatomy**: Deep muscle. Most part of the muscle underlies the extensor carpi radialis and extensor digitorum communis muscle at the proximal forearm supinated position.
- **Origin**: Lateral supracondylar, ulnar, and radius ligaments of elbow joints.
- **Insertion**: Proximal radial lateral side.
- **Function**: Supination forearm.
- **Motor point (MP)**: Proximal one-fourth point (MP) between the lateral condyle (A) and ulnar styloid process (B).
- **Injection tip**: At sitting or supine position, keep the forearm in pronated and flexed position. Supinator solely supinates the forearm at this position. If fingers extension is noted, the needle is located in the extensor digitorum communis. Push the needle deeper until to see supination of the forearm.

Hand

5.1 Abductor pollicis brevis

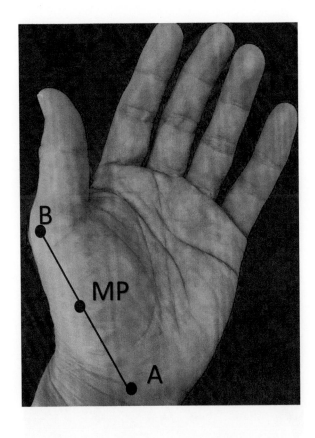

- **Surface anatomy**: Most superficial layer of thenar muscles and lies most radial side.
- **Origin**: Transverse carpal ligament and radial carpal bones.
- **Insertion**: Radial base of proximal phalanx of thumb.
- **Function**: Abduction thumb at carpometacarpal and metacarpophalangeal joints of the thumb.
- **Motor point (MP)**: Midpoint between the midpoint of the wrist joint (A) and the lateral part of the thumb metacarpophalangeal joint (B).
- **Injection tip**: At forearm fully supinated and hand opening position, insert needle to the motor point (remember this is a superficial muscle). Make sure the thumb abduction not flexion or opposition.

5.2 Opponens pollicis

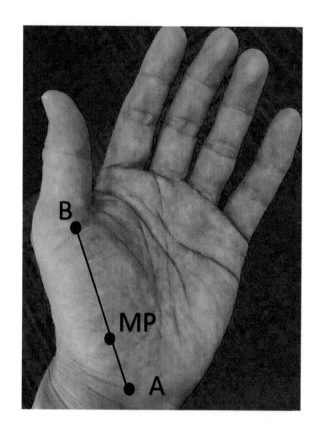

- **Surface anatomy**: Mostly underlies abductor pollicis brevis.
- **Origin**: Transverse carpal ligament and trapezium.
- **Insertion**: Metacarpal bone of thumb.
- **Function**: Flexion and abduction the thumb at carpometacarpal joint.
- **Motor point (MP)**: One-third (close to wrist) between midpoint of wrist (A) and the midpoint of the palmar digital crease of the thumb (B)[15].
- **Injection tip**: At forearm fully supinated and hand opening position, insert needle to the motor point. Make sure the thumb moves toward to the little finger.

5.3 Flexor pollicis brevis

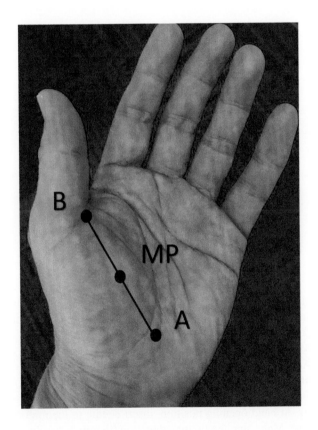

- **Surface anatomy**: One of thenar muscles superficially and distally located with two (superficial and deep) parts.
- **Origin**: Trapezium and flexor retinaculum.

- **Insertion**: Proximal phalanx of thumb.
- **Function**: Flex thumb at MP joint.
- **Motor point (MP)**: Midpoint between the distal connection (A) of the thenar and hypothenar eminence and medial side of the thumb metacarpophalangeal joint (B).
- **Injection tip**: At forearm fully supinated and hand opening position, insert needle to the motor point (remember this has both superficial and deep layers). Make sure the thumb flexion at metacarpophalangeal joint. If the needle is in the adductor pollicis, the thumb adduction is seen.

5.4 Adductor pollicis

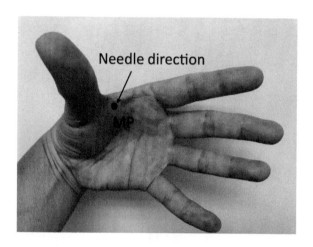

- **Surface anatomy**: Volar side of space between thumb and index finger
- **Origin**: Transverse part: third metacarpal. Oblique part: second and third meta-carpals, trapezoid, and capitate.
- **Insertion**: Medial side of proximal phalanx of thumb.
- **Function**: Adduction thumb at carpometacarpal joint.
- **Motor point (MP)**: Midpoint of the volar side of ridge (skin fold) between the thumb and index finger.
- **Injection tip**: At hand opening position, insert needle to the motor point toward the thumb base. Make sure the thumb adduction (thumb moves toward the index finger). If thumb flexion at metacarpophalangeal joint is noted, the needle is not in the adductor pollicis, but in the flexor pollicis brevis.

5.5 **Flexor digiti minimi brevis**

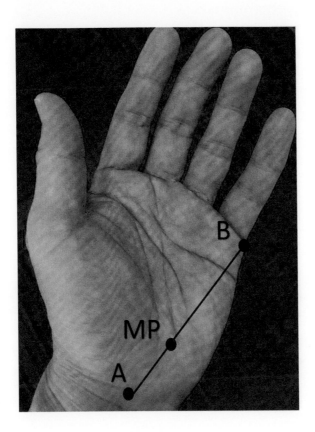

- **Surface anatomy**: Inner side of hypothenar muscles.
- **Origin**: Hamate.
- **Insertion**: Proximal phalanx of little finger.
- **Function**: Flex little finger at metacarpophalangeal joint.
- **Motor point (MP)**: Proximal one-third point between the midpoint of the wrist crease (A) and the ulnar side end of the little finger metacarpophalangeal joint (B).
- **Injection tip**: At forearm fully supinated and hand opening position, insert needle to the motor point. Make sure the little finger flexion.

5.6 Adductor digiti minimi

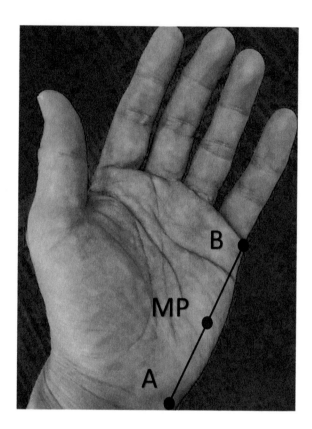

- **Surface anatomy**: Outer side hypothenar muscles.
- **Origin**: Pisiform and flexor retinaculum.
- **Insertion**: Proximal phalanx of little finger.
- **Function**: Abduction little finger.
- **Motor point (MP)**: Midpoint of wrist ulnar end (A) and little finger meta-carpophalangeal joint ulnar side (B).
- **Injection tip**: At forearm fully supinated and hand opening position, insert needle to the motor point. Make sure the little finger abduction.

5.7 **Lumbricals**

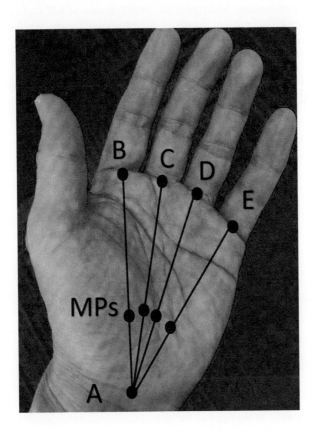

- **Surface anatomy**: Small and narrow. Deeply located between inter-metacarpal bones. Four muscles (from radial side to ulnar side). The first and second lumbricals are located along the radial side of the second and third metacarpal bone. The third and fourth are between fourth and fifth metacarpal bone.
- **Origin**: Flexor digitorum profundus tendons.
- **Insertion**: Extensor expansions.
- **Function**: Flexion metacarpophalangeal joints and extension proximal interphalangeal and distal interphalangeal joints.

- **Motor point (MP)**: Proximal one-third points (MPs) between center of wrist crease (A) and each metacarpophalangeal joints (B-E).
- **Injection tip**: At forearm fully supinated and hand opening, insert needle through palm. Painful procedure. Make sure the finger flexion at MP and extension the proximal interphalangeal and the distal interphalangeal joints (each finger moves corresponding to each lumbricals).

5.8 Dorsal interossei (the first)

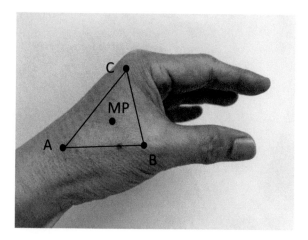

- **Surface anatomy**: Superficial in the first interdigital web (dorsal aspect).
- **Origin**: On the radial side of the second metacarpal and the proximal half of the ulnar side of the first metacarpal.
- **Insertion**: Proximal phalanx of index finger and extensor expansions
- **Function**: abduct index finger.
- **Motor point (MP)**: Center of the triangle (A: anatomical snuff box, B: thumb metacarpophalangeal joint, C: index finger metacarpophalangeal joint).
- **Injection tip**: At forearm fully pronated, extend wrist 30−40 degrees. Insert needle through the dorsum of the hand. Make sure the index finger abduction.

5.9 **Dorsal interossei (second- fourth)**

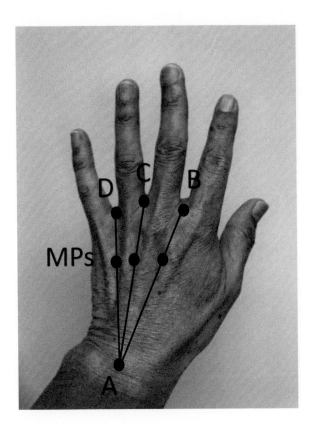

- **Surface anatomy**: Located between inter-metacarpal bones (dorsal aspect)
- **Origin**: Metacarpals.
- **Insertion**: Proximal phalanx of fingers and extensor expansions.
- **Function**: Abduct finger(s).
- **Motor point (MP)**: Distal one-third from center of wrist creases (A, dorsum) and each interdigital spaces (B-D).
- **Injection tip**: At forearm fully pronated, palpate each metacarpal bone (2nd to 5th) and insert needle between the bones through the dorsum of the hand. Make sure the finger abduction (each finger abduction corresponding to each dorsal interossei).

5.10 Palmar interossei

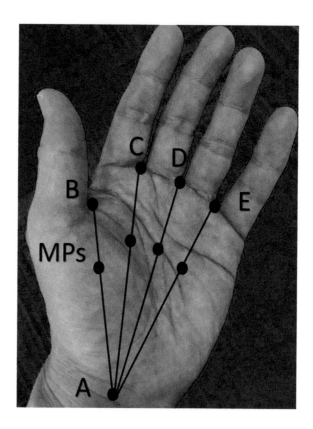

- **Surface anatomy**: Small and narrow four muscles (first to fourth). Located deep along the metacarpal bones (palmar aspect); first and second along the ulnar side of first and second metacarpal bone respectively. Third and fourth along the radial side of the fourth and fifth metacarpal bone respectively.
- **Origin**: Metacarpals.
- **Insertion**: Extensor expansions.
- **Function**: Adduct finger(s).
- **Motor point (MP)**: 4 motor points for each muscle.
  - first palmar interosseous: distal one-third between mid-wrist (A) and thumb metacarpophalangeal joint ulnar side (B).
  - second palmar interosseous: distal one-third between mid-wrist (A) and second interdigital space (C).
  - third & fourth palmar interosseous: distal one-third from mid-wrist (A) and third and fourth interdigital space respectively (D & E).
- **Injection tip**: At forearm fully supinated, insert needle between the metacarpal bones through the palm. Make sure the finger adduction (each finger abduction corresponding to each dorsal interossei).

Upper leg

6.1 Iliopsoas

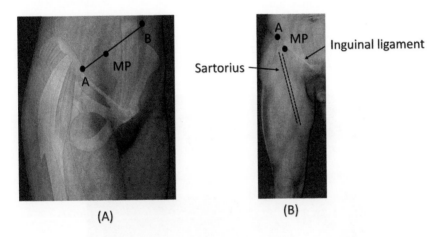

(A)   (B)

(A) From Moses KP, Nava P, Banks J, Petersen D. Chapter 41 - Hip Joint, Atlas of Clinical Gross Anatomy. 2ⁿᵈ ed. Elsevier/Saunders; 2013; (B) From Moses KP, Nava P, Banks J, Petersen D. Chapter 40 - Anteromedial Thigh, Atlas of Clinical Gross Anatomy. 2ⁿᵈ ed. Elsevier/Saunders; 2013

- **Surface anatomy**: Two (iliacus and psoas) muscles are deep in the abdominal cavity and superficial distal to the inguinal ligament and medial to the Sartorius muscle.
- **Origin**: Iliac fossa for iliacus and lumbar spine for psoas muscles.
- **Insertion**: Lesser trochanter of the femur.
- **Function**: Flexion hip.
- **Motor point (MP)**: Three different techniques.
  1. Suprainguinal approach (Fig. A)[16–18]: Distal one-third point between anterior superior iliac spine (A) and umbilicus (B). At supine position, press down medial side of anterior superior iliac spine with fingers and then pushing away

internal organs medially. Insert needle slowly until hit the bone (iliac bone). Then slowly pull the needle back.

2. Infrainguinal approach (Fig. B)[18,19]: At supine positon, using ultrasound, identify the muscle over the femoral head or at the inferiomedial to the ASIS (A). At this site, femoral nerve is close to medial side. Insert needle cranially (but less likely motor point targeted).

3. Posterior approach[20]: At side lying or prone position, using ultrasound or CT, identify the muscle.

• **Injection tip**: For suprainguinal approach, a long injection needle is needed. Push the motor point with fingers as much as deep down and medially to avoid internal organ puncture. Then slowly insert a needle down to hit the iliac bone. Then slowly pull back the needle with electrical stimulation. If the needle is close to the femoral nerve, then strong knee extension is noted. If needle is placed superficially, then abdominal muscles contract.

6.2 Tensor fascia lata

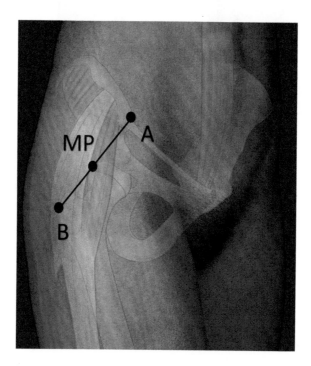

From Moses KP, Nava P, Banks J, Petersen D. Chapter 41 - Hip Joint, Atlas of Clinical Gross Anatomy. 2nd ed. Elsevier/Saunders; 2013

- **Surface anatomy**: Superficial muscles from lateral side of ASIS to the lateral knee.
- **Origin**: Iliac crest.
- **Insertion**: Iliotibial band.
- **Function**: Internal rotation and flexion hip.
- **Motor point**: Midpoint between anterior superior iliac spine (A) and greater trochanter (B).
- **Injection tip**: At supine, put the thumb at the anterior superior iliac spine and middle finger at the greater trochanter, the index finger tip will be placed on the motor point. The muscle is bulged with internal rotation of the hip at the motor point.

6.3 **Gluteus maximus**

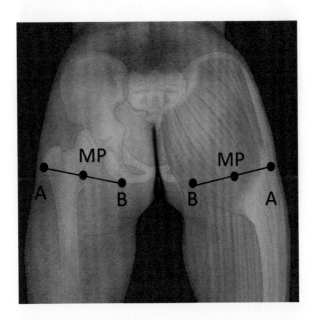

From Moses KP, Nava P, Banks J, Petersen D. Chapter 36 - Pelvic Girdle, Atlas of Clinical Gross Anatomy. 2nd ed.
Elsevier/Saunders; 2013

- **Surface anatomy**: The largest and superficial muscle from the buttock.
- **Origin**: Posterior ilium and sacrum.
- **Insertion**: Greater tuberosity of femur.
- **Function**: Extension and external rotation hip.

- **Motor point (MP)**: Midpoint between the greater trochanter (A) and the ischial tuberosity (B).
- **Injection tip**: At prone with slight hip abduction, insert the needle slowly into deep. If sciatic nerve is stimulated, pull back the needle. The sciatic nerve is deep to the muscle.

6.4 Gluteus medius

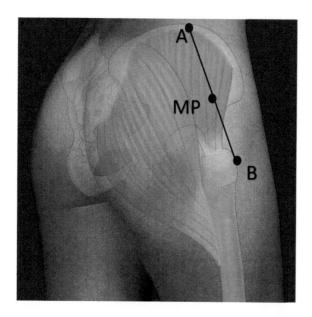

From Moses KP, Nava P, Banks J, Petersen D. Chapter 41 - Hip Joint, Atlas of Clinical Gross Anatomy. 2ⁿᵈ ed.
Elsevier/Saunders; 2013

- **Surface anatomy**: Upper right quadrant of the buttock (partially covered with gluteus maximus in the lower part).
- **Origin**: Posterior ilium.
- **Insertion**: Greater trochanter of femur.
- **Function**: Abduction hip.
- **Motor point**: Midpoint between upper most iliac crest (A) and greater trochanter (B).
- **Injection tip**: At prone with slight hip abduction or at side lying position.

6.5 **Gluteus minimus**

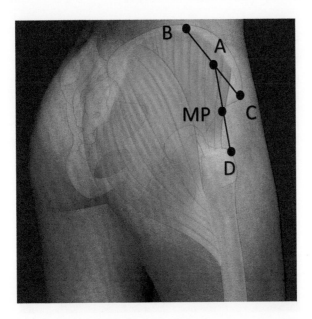

*From Moses KP, Nava P, Banks J, Petersen D. Chapter 41 - Hip Joint, Atlas of Clinical Gross Anatomy. 2ⁿᵈ ed.
Elsevier/Saunders; 2013*

- **Surface anatomy**: Difficult to be identified superficially because most of the muscle is covered by gluteus maximus and medius in the upper right quadrant of the buttock.
- **Origin**: outer surface of the ilium (between the anterior and inferior gluteal line) and he margin of the greater sciatic notch.
- **Insertion**: Greater trochanter of femur.
- **Function**: Abduction hip.
- **Motor point**: Midpoint between the midpoint (A), which is in the middle of top of iliac crest (B) and superior anterior iliac spine (C), and greater trochanter (D).
- **Injection tip**: At prone with slight hip abduction or at side lying position. MP is deep (through gluteus medius).

6.6 Deep hip external rotators (piriformis, gemellus, obturators, quadrutus femoris)

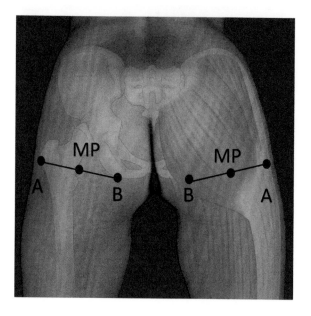

From Moses KP, Nava P, Banks J, Petersen D. Chapter 36 - Pelvic Girdle, Atlas of Clinical Gross Anatomy. 2nd ed. Elsevier/Saunders; 2013

- **Surface anatomy**: Small and deep muscles of the lower lateral quadrant buttock (covered with gluteus maximus).
- **Origin**: Posterior ilium, ischium, and sacrum.
- **Insertion**: Greater trochanter and intertrochanteric crest of femur.
- **Function**: External rotation hip.
- **Motor point (MP)**: Midpoint between greater trochanter (A) and ischial tuberosity (B) (superficially same point as the gluteus maximus MP but deeper).
- **Injection tip**: At prone with slight hip abduction, since the muscle is deep, insert the needle slowly into deep (lateral to the sciatic nerve).

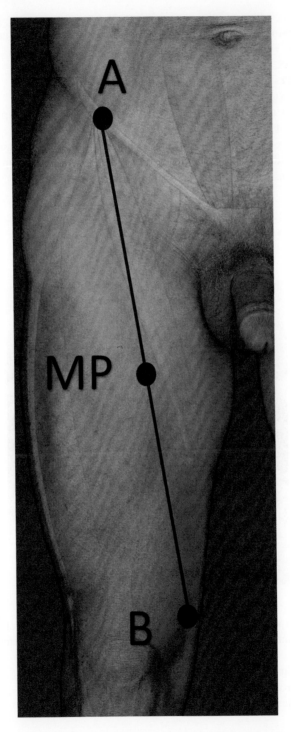

From Moses KP, Nava P, Banks J, Petersen D. Chapter 40 - Anteromedial Thigh, Atlas of Clinical Gross Anatomy. 2nd ed. Elsevier/Saunders; 2013

- **Surface anatomy**: Superficial muscles from anterior superior iliac spine to the medial knee. Forms lateral border of Scarpa's (femoral) triangle.
- **Origin**: ASIS.
- **Insertion**: Pes anserius.
- **Function**: External rotation, flexion, and abduction hip.
- **Motor point (MP)**: Midpoint from the anterior superior iliac spine (A) to the medial side of the knee (B).
- **Injection tip**: Scarpa's or femoral triangle is formed by inguinal ligament superiorly, adductor longus medially, and Sartorius laterally. At supine and slight hip abduction, the muscle is superficial.

6.8 Pectineus

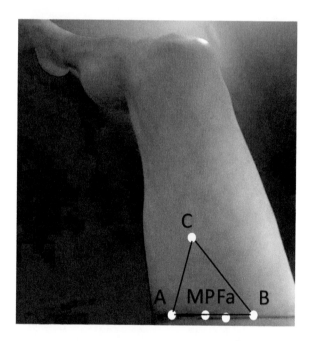

- **Surface anatomy**: Most superficial and lateral hip adductor muscle from medial pubic bone and located between adductor longus (medial) and femoral artery (lateral).
- **Origin**: Medial pubis.
- **Insertion**: Proximal femur medial side.
- **Function**: Flexion and adduction hip.

- **Motor point (MP)**: Between the medial point (A) of Scarpa's (femoral) triangle (ABC) and femoral artery (Fa, palpate the artery to avoid the artery puncture).
- **Injection tip**: At supine with slight hip abduction, the motor point is located superficially. Obturator nerve is stimulated if the needle goes too deep and medially, and femoral nerve is stimulated if the needle goes too laterally.

6.9 Adductor longus

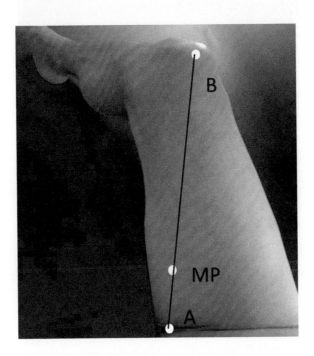

- **Surface anatomy**: Superficial muscles from inguinal groove to the mid-portion of the thigh medial side. Forms medial border of Scarpa's (femoral) triangle.
- **Origin**: Pubis.
- **Insertion**: Medial side of the middle part of femur.
- **Function**: Adduction hip.
- **Motor point (MP)**[17,21]: Proximal one-fourth between the medial point of Scarpa's (femoral) triangle (A) and mid-portion of the patella upper pole (B).
- **Injection tip**: At supine with slight hip abduction, the motor point is located deeply.

6.10 Adductor magnus

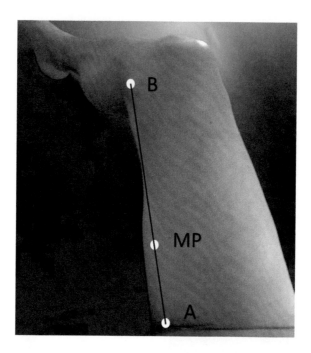

- **Surface anatomy**: Mostly underlies adductor longus and brevis in the medial side (deep).
- **Origin**: Pubic tuberosity.
- **Insertion**: Medial side of the middle and distal part of femur.
- **Function**: Hip adduction.
- **Motor point (MP)**[17,21]: Proximal one-third between the medial point of Scarpa's (femoral) triangle (A) and medial side of the knee (B).
- **Injection tip**: At supine with slight hip abduction, the motor point of the muscle is more distal and medial to the adductor longus motor point.

6.11 **Adductor brevis**

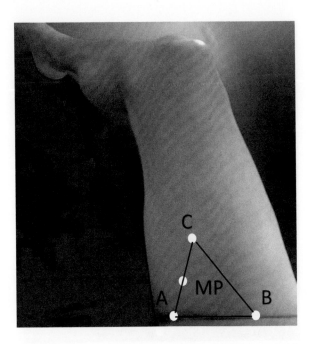

- **Surface anatomy**: Deep muscles from inguinal groove to the upper one-third portion of the thigh medial side (mostly covered with pectineus and adductor longus).
- **Origin**: Pubis.
- **Insertion**: Medial side of the middle part of femur.
- **Function**: Hip adduction.
- **Motor point (MP)**[17,21]: Midpoint between the medial point (A) and distal point (C) of Scarpa's (femoral) triangle (ABC).
- **Injection tip**: At supine with slight hip abduction, the motor point is located deeper and more lateral to the adductor longus motor point.

6.12 **Gracilis**

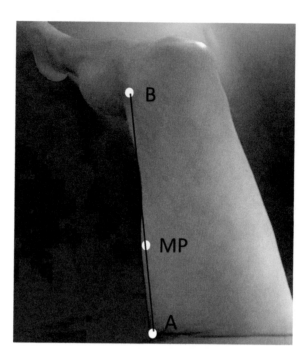

- **Surface anatomy**: Most medial part of thigh (thin long narrow muscle) between adductor longus and medial hamstring at the origin and between sartorius and medial hamstring at the insertion.
- **Origin**: Ischiopubic ramus.
- **Insertion**: Medial side of knee (pes anserius).
- **Function**: Adduction, flexion, and medial rotation hip.
- **Motor point (MP)**[22]: Proximal one-third between medial inguinal (A) and medial knee (B).
- **Injection tip**: At supine with hip abduction, the motor point is almost same as adductor magnus MP, but it is located more superficially and more medially to the adductor magnus MP.

6.13 Rectus femoris

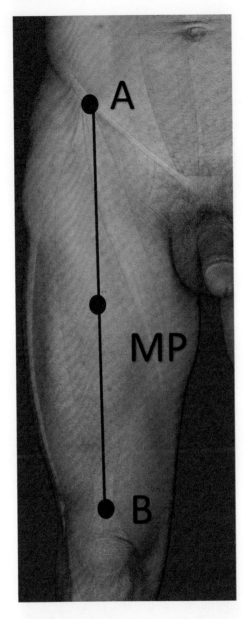

- **Surface anatomy**: Mid part of anterior thigh between sartorious and tensor fascia lata.
- **Origin**: Anterior superior iliac spine.
- **Insertion**: Patella tendon.
- **Function**: Extension knee and flexion hip.
- **Motor point (MP)**[23–25]: Midpoint between anterior superior iliac spine (A) and patella proximal end (B).

- **Injection tip**: At supine with slight hip abduction, the motor point is located superficially.

6.14 Vastus lateralis

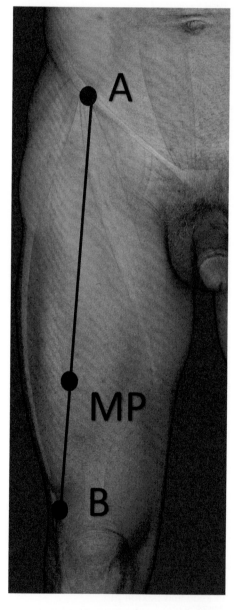

From Moses KP, Nava P, Banks J, Petersen D. Chapter 40 - Anteromedial Thigh, Atlas of Clinical Gross Anatomy.
2nd ed. Elsevier/Saunders; 2013

- **Surface anatomy**: Lateral part of lower anterolateral thigh.
- **Origin**: Greater trochanter of femur.
- **Insertion**: Patella tendon.
- **Function**: Extension knee.
- **Motor point (MP)**[23–25]: Lower one-third point between anterior superior iliac spine (A) and patella lateral end (B).
- **Injection tip**: At supine with slight hip abduction, the motor point is located between lateral border of the rectus femoris and medial border of the iliotibial band.

6.15 Vastus medialis

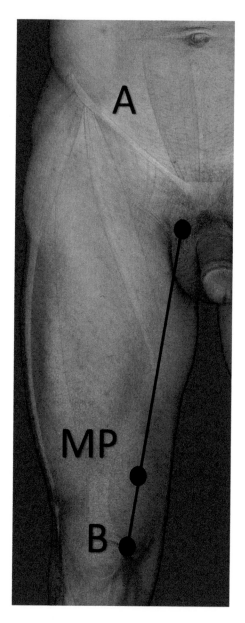

From Moses KP, Nava P, Banks J, Petersen D. Chapter 40 - Anteromedial Thigh, Atlas of Clinical Gross Anatomy.
2nd ed. Elsevier/Saunders; 2013

- **Surface anatomy**: Medial part of lower anteromedial thigh.
- **Origin**: Intertrochanteric line of femur.
- **Insertion**: Patella tendon.

- **Function**: Extension knee.
- **Motor point (MP)**[23–25]: Lower one-fourth point between medial inguinal ligament (A) and medial patella (B).
- **Injection tip**: At supine with slight hip abduction, the motor point is located between lateral border of rectus femoris and medial border of iliotibial band.

6.16 Vastus intermedius

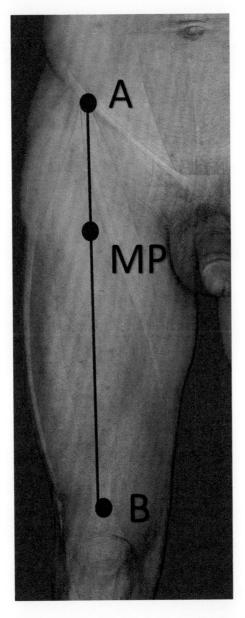

From Moses KP, Nava P, Banks J, Petersen D. Chapter 40 - Anteromedial Thigh, Atlas of Clinical Gross Anatomy.
2nd ed. Elsevier/Saunders; 2013

- **Surface anatomy**: Deep muscle underlying rectus femoris and bordered medially by vastus medialis and laterally by vastus laterally. Difficult to identify superficially.
- **Origin**: Anterolateral aspect of proximal femur.
- **Insertion**: Patella tendon.
- **Function**: Extension knee.
- **Motor point (MP)**[23–25]: Upper one-third between and anterior superior iliac spine (A) and upper patella (B).
- **Injection tip**: At supine with slight hip abduction, since the muscle is in deep, the MP is in deep (hit the femur with the needle, and then slowly pull back).

6.17 Hamstring (medial)

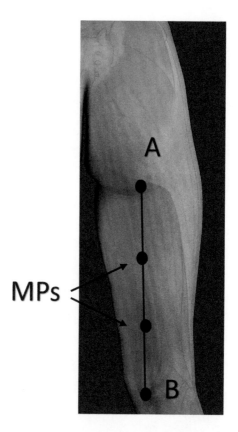

From Moses KP, Nava P, Banks J, Petersen D. Chapter 42 - Gluteal Region/Posterior Thigh, Atlas of Clinical Gross Anatomy. 2nd ed. Elsevier/Saunders; 2013

- **Surface anatomy**: Medial hamstrings are composed of semimembranosus and semitendiosus.
- **Origin**: Ischial tuberosity.
- **Insertion**: Medial proximal tibia.
- **Function**: Flexion knee and extension hip.
- **Motor point (MP)**[23,26]: Mostly distributed between proximal and distal one-third point between ischial tuberosity (A) and medial popliteal crease (B). If two injection sites are needed, the proximal and the distal on third between A and B will be the targets.
- **Injection tip**: Individual variation is common. Keep the needle medial side of the muscle. If needle is close to the sciatic nerve, movements of toes and ankles will be noticed. Sciatic nerve is located between medial and lateral hamstrings.

6.18 Hamstring (lateral)

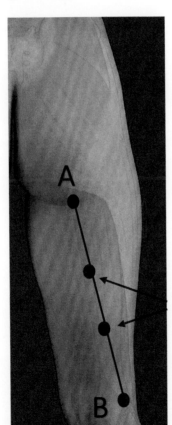

From Moses KP, Nava P, Banks J, Petersen D. Chapter 42 - Gluteal Region/Posterior Thigh, Atlas of Clinical Gross Anatomy. 2nd ed. Elsevier/Saunders; 2013

- **Surface anatomy**: Lateral hamstrings are composed of biceps femoris short and long head.
- **Origin**: Ischial tuberosity (long head) and femur (short head).
- **Insertion**: Lateral proximal tibia.
- **Function**: Flexion knee and extension hip.
- **Motor point (MP)**[23,26]: Mostly distributed between proximal and distal one-third between ischial tuberosity (A) and lateral popliteal crease (B). If two injection sites are needed, the proximal and the distal point will be the targets.
- **Injection tip**: Individual variation is common. Keep the needle medial side of the muscle. If needle is close to the sciatic nerve, movements of toes and ankles will be noticed. Sciatic nerve is located between medial and lateral hamstrings.

Lower leg

7.1 Gastrocnemius (medial)

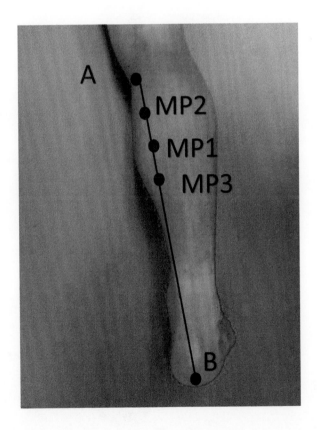

- **Surface anatomy**: Prominent upper half of calf medial side.
- **Origin**: Medial condyle of femur.

Botulinum Neurotoxin. https://doi.org/10.1016/B978-0-323-69715-6.00021-1

- **Insertion**: Calcaneus (Achilles tendon).
- **Function**: Plantar flexion ankle and flexion knee.
- **Motor point (MP)**[27–29]: Just proximal of the most prominent muscle belly (MP1), about proximal one-fourth between medial popliteal crease (A) and heel (B). If multiple injections are needed, MP2 (between MP1 and A) and MP3 (same distance from MP1 to MP2 distally) are recommended.
- **Injection tip**: If needle is deep close to the tibial nerve, movements of toes will be noticed. Medial gastrocnemius MP3 is proximal to soleus MP3.

7.2 Gastrocnemius (lateral)

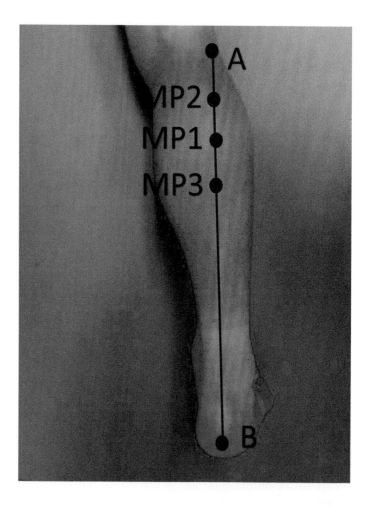

- **Surface anatomy**: Prominent upper half of calf lateral side.
- **Origin**: Lateral condyle of femur.

- **Insertion**: Calcaneus (Achilles tendon).
- **Function**: Plantar flexion ankle and flexion knee.
- **Motor point**:[27–29] Just proximal of the most prominent muscle belly (MP1) about proximal one-fourth between lateral popliteal crease (A) and heel (B). If multiple injections are needed, MP2 (between MP1 and A) and MP3 (same distance from MP1 to MP2 distally) are recommended.
- **Injection tip**: If needle is deep close to the tibial nerve, movements of toes will be noticed. Medial gastrocnemius MP3 is very close to soleus MP1, but more superficial than soleus MP1.

7.3 Soleus

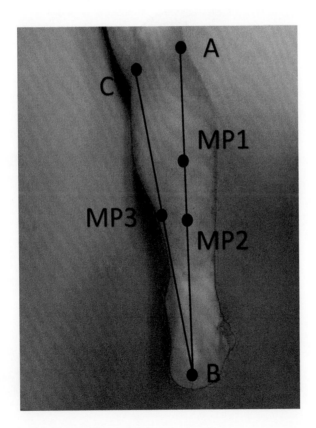

- **Surface anatomy**: Proximally covered by gastrocnemius muscles (deep), and superficial distal to half of the calf.
- **Origin**: Fibula and medial proximal tibia.
- **Insertion**: Calcaneus (Achilles tendon).

- **Function**: Plantar flexion ankle.
- **Motor points (MPs)**[27–29]: 3 MPs.
  1. MP1: proximal one-third between lateral popliteal crease (A) and heel (B) (deep).
  2. MP2: midpoint between lateral popliteal crease (A) and heel (B) (superficial).
  3. MP3: midpoint between medial popliteal crease (C) and heel (B) (superficial).
- **Injection tip**: If toes moves, the needle is close to tibial nerve. MP 1 is in deep (under gastrocnemius lateral head). MP2 &3 are superficial.

7.4 Peroneus longus

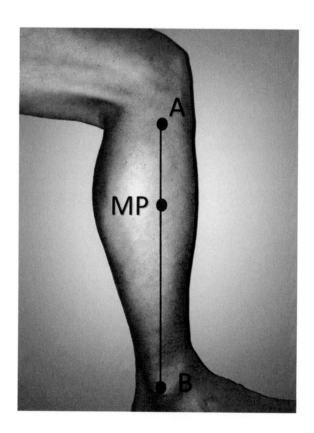

- **Surface anatomy**: Proximally it lies between tibialis anterior and gastrocnemius lateral head.
- **Origin**: Upper lateral fibula.
- **Insertion**: First metatarsal and medial cuneiform.
- **Function**: Plantar flexion ankle and foot eversion.

- **Motor point (MP)**[27]: Proximal one-third between the fibular head (A) and lateral malleolus (B).
- **Injection tip**: If needle is in tibialis anterior, foot inversion is seen. If the needle is in the right place, the peroneus longus tendon movement is seen at the behind of the lateral malleolus.

7.5 Peroneus brevis

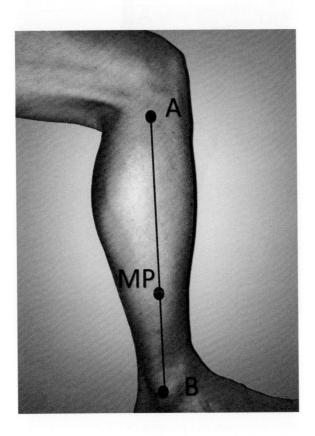

- **Surface anatomy**: In the lower half lateral aspect of the lower leg, it lies underneath the peroneus longus and becomes superficial at the distal part (motor point area).
- **Origin**: Lower fibula.
- **Insertion**: Fifth metatarsal dorsum.
- **Function**: Eversion foot and plantar flexion ankle.
- **Motor point (MP)**: Distal one-third between the fibular head (A) and lateral malleolus (B).
- **Injection tip**: The peroneus brevis tendon runs behind the lateral malleolus (same as the peroneus longus).

7.6 Peroneus tertius

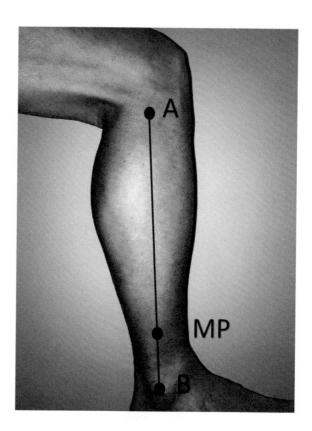

- **Surface anatomy**: Difficult to identify superficially. It is located between peroneus brevis (laterally) and the extensor digitorum longus tendons (medially).
- **Origin**: Distal fibula.
- **Insertion**: Fifth metatarsal.
- **Function**: Dorsiflexion ankle and eversion foot.
- **Motor point (MP)**: Lower one-quarter between lateral malleolus (A) and fibular head (B) (between the peroneus brevis and the extensor digitorum longus tendon).
- **Injection tip**: It is difficult to find the motor point of this small and thin muscle. If tendon movement behind the lateral malleolus is seen, the needle is in the peroneus brevis. If needle is in the right place, lateral foot dorsiflexion (see function above) is seen.

7.7 Tibialis anterior

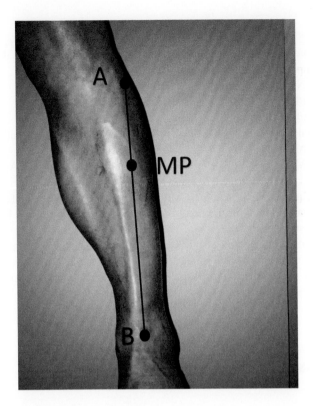

- **Surface anatomy**: Anterolateral part of the lower leg along the tibia.
- **Origin**: Upper lateral tibia.
- **Insertion**: First metatarsal and medial cuneiform.
- **Function**: Dorsiflexion ankle and foot inversion.
- **Motor point (MP)**: proximal one-third between the tibial lateral condyle (A) and mid-point of ankle dorsum (B).

7.8 Tibialis posterior

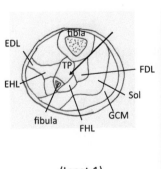

(Inset 1)

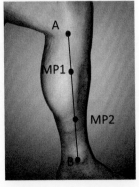

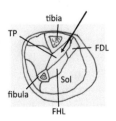

(Inset 2)

- **Surface anatomy**: Difficult to identify superficially because this is deep muscle.
- **Origin**: Upper posterior tibia and fibula.
- **Insertion**: Navicular and medial cuneiform.
- **Function**: Plantar flexion ankle and foot inversion.
- **Motor points (2 MPs)**[30,31]:
  1) Proximal (MP1): proximal one-third between tibial medial condyle (A) and medial malleolus (B). MP 1 is really deep (see Inset 1).
  2) Distal (MP2): distal one-third between tibial medial condyle (A) and medial malleolus (B). MP2 is not deep (see Inset 2).
- **Injection tip**: For MP1, at supine and knee flexion position, palpate the gap between tibia and medial gastrocnemius muscle. Inset needle (arrow) from medial to lateral just underneath the tibial bone parallel to intermalleolus axis. If toe flexion is noted, the needle does not reach the tibialis posterior yet and if great toe extension is noted, the needle is too deep (Inset 1). For MP2, same position as for MP1, insert needle (arrow) just as the MP1 (medial to lateral and parallel to intermalleolus axis). If toe flexion is noted, the needle is not reach the MP2 yet (Inset 2).

7.9 Extensor digitorum longus

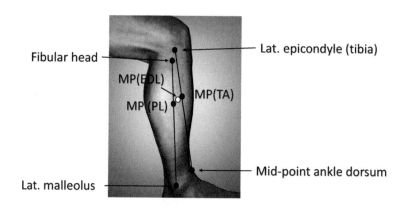

- **Surface anatomy**: Superficial between tibialis anterior (medially) and peroneus longus (laterally).
- **Origin**: Anterolateral tibia.
- **Insertion**: Dorsum of middle and distal phalanges of lateral four toes.
- **Function**: Extension lateral four toes.

- **Motor point (MP)**: Between the motor points of the peroneus longus muscles (A, see 7-4) and tibialis anterior (B, see 7-7).
- **Injection tip**: Be sure to confirm extension of the lateral four toes only. If the needle is in deep, it may reach extensor halluces longus (great toe extension).

7.10 Extensor hallucis longus

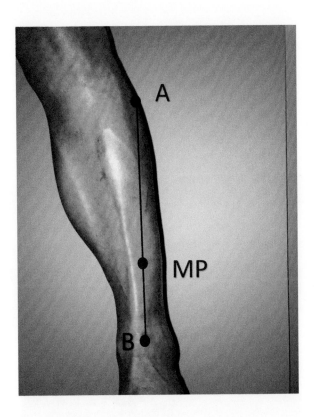

- **Surface anatomy**: It lies deep to the extensor digitorum longus and between the tibialis anterior and the peroneus longus at the mid part of the lower leg. The tendon of extensor hallucis longus is seen at the ankle between the tendons of the extensor digitorum longus and tibialis anterior.
- **Origin**: Middle portion of fibula.
- **Insertion**: Dorsum of distal phalanges of the great toe.
- **Function**: Extension the great toe.

- **Motor point (MP)**: Between the tendons of the tibialis anterior (medial) and the extensor digitorum longus (lateral) at the lower one-third point from fibular head (A) to mid-point of ankle dorsum(B).
- **Injection tip**: Isolated extension of the great toe is noticed if the needle is in the motor point.

7.11 Flexor digitorum longus

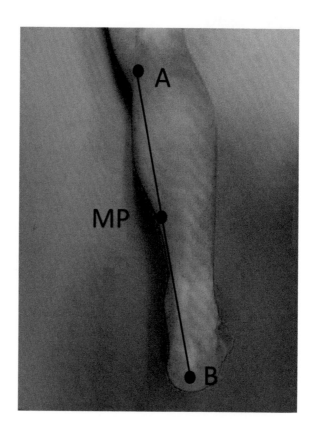

- **Surface anatomy**: Difficult to be identified, because it is posterior to tibia and covered with heel cord muscles.
- **Origin**: Proximal one-third point of the tibia posteriorly.
- **Insertion**: Base of the distal phalanges of the lateral four toes.
- **Function**: Flexion lateral four toes.

- **Motor point (MP)**: Midpoint between medial end of popliteal crease (A) and heel (B). MP is similar spot for soleus medial side motor point (MP3, see 7-3), but deeper than soleus MP3.
- **Injection tip**: The motor point is in deep. If needle is not enough deep, soleus contraction can be seen instead of the lateral four toes flexion. If needle is in too deep, tibialis posterior contraction can be seen (see 7-8, MP2).

7.12 **Flexor hallucis longus**

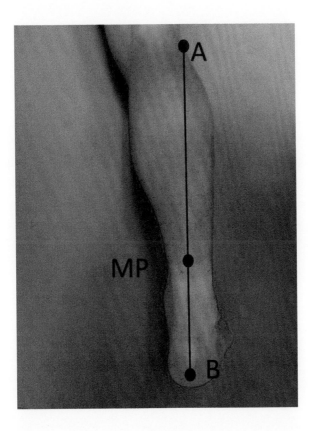

- **Surface anatomy**: Difficult to be identified, because it is deep to the heel cord muscles. It goes down between peroneus and heel cord muscles.
- **Origin**: Middle one-third of the fibula posteriorly.
- **Insertion**: Base of the distal phalanges of the great toe.

- **Function**: Flexion great toe.
- **Motor point (MP)**: Lower one-third between the lateral end of popliteal crease (A) and heel (B).
- **Injection tip**: The motor point is in deep. If needle is not enough deep, soleus contraction can be seen instead of the great toe flexion.

Foot

8.1 Abductor hallucis

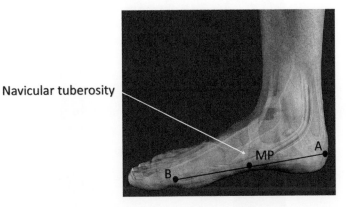

Navicular tuberosity

From Moses KP, Nava P, Banks J, Petersen D. Chapter 47 - Foot, Atlas of Clinical Gross Anatomy. 2nd ed.
Elsevier/Saunders; 2013

- **Surface anatomy**: Medial side of the foot.
- **Origin**: Tuberosity of calcaneus and flexor retinaculum.
- **Insertion**: Base of the medial side of the proximal phalanges of the great toe.
- **Function**: Abduction the great toe.
- **Motor point (MP)**[32,33]: Midpoint (just inferior to the navicular tuberosity) between heel end (A) and medial side of first metatarsal bone (B).
- **Injection tip**: The motor point is superficial.

Botulinum Neurotoxin. https://doi.org/10.1016/B978-0-323-69715-6.00020-X

8.2 Adductor hallucis (transvers)

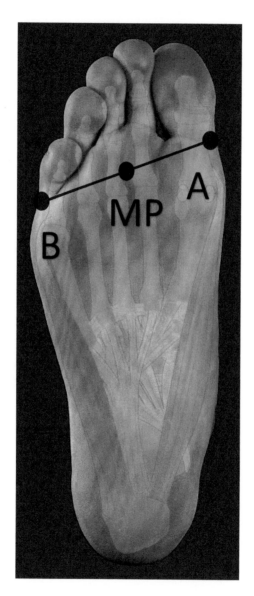

From Moses KP, Nava P, Banks J, Petersen D. Chapter 47 - Foot, Atlas of Clinical Gross Anatomy. 2nd ed. Elsevier/Saunders; 2013

- **Surface anatomy**: The deepest muscle of the foot intrinsic muscles (the third layer muscles).
- **Origin**: Metatarsophalangeal joints of the lateral three toes (third to fifth).

- **Insertion**: Lateral side of the base of the proximal phalanges of the great toe.
- **Function**: Adduction the great toe.
- **Motor point (MP)**: Midpoint between medial base of the great toe (A) and the lateral base of the fifth toe (B).
- **Injection tip**: Approach from the sole.

8.3 Adductor hallucis (oblique)

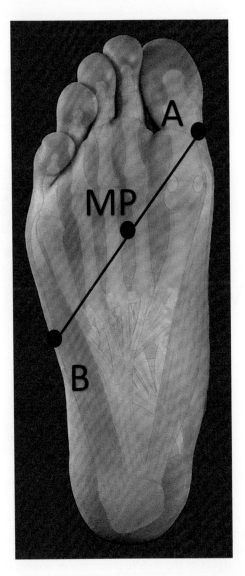

From Moses KP, Nava P, Banks J, Petersen D. Chapter 47 - Foot, Atlas of Clinical Gross Anatomy. 2nd ed.
Elsevier/Saunders; 2013

- **Surface anatomy**: The deepest muscle of the foot intrinsic muscles (the third layer muscles). Oblique head is deep to flexor digitorum brevis muscle and it is difficult to be identified superficially.
- **Origin**: Middle three metatarsal bones.
- **Insertion**: Lateral side of the base of the proximal phalanges of the great toe.
- **Function**: Adduction the great toe.
- **Motor point (MP)**: Midpoint between medial base of the great toe (A) and the lateral head of the fifth metatarsal bone (B).

8.4 Flexor digitorum brevis

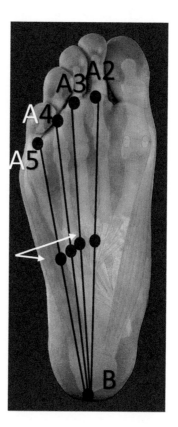

From Moses KP, Nava P, Banks J, Petersen D. Chapter 47 - Foot, Atlas of Clinical Gross Anatomy. 2nd ed.
Elsevier/Saunders; 2013

- **Surface anatomy**: The muscles are one of the most superficial foot intrinsic muscles (the first layer).
- **Origin**: Calcaneus base.
- **Insertion**: Plantar aspect of the middle phalanges of second through fifth toes.
- **Function**: Flexion proximal interphalangeal joints of toes (second to fifth).

- **Motor points (MPs)**: Midpoints (MP2-5) between bases of the toes (A2—A5) and heel end (B).
- **Injection tip**: The muscle is superficial and lies between abductor halluces medially and abductor digiti minimi laterally at the middle of the plantar foot. If the needle is located in deep, great toe adduction can be seen.

8.5 Abductor digiti minimi

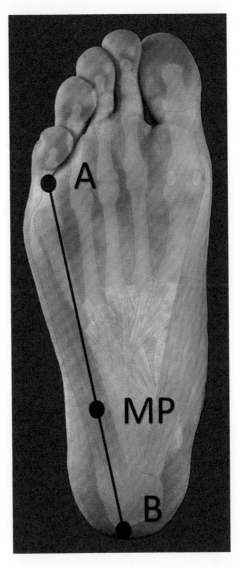

From Moses KP, Nava P, Banks J, Petersen D. Chapter 47 - Foot, Atlas of Clinical Gross Anatomy. 2nd ed.
Elsevier/Saunders; 2013

- **Surface anatomy**: The muscles is one of the most superficial foot intrinsic muscles (the first layer). It lies in the posterior half of the foot lateral portion.
- **Origin**: Calcaneal tuberosity and plantar aponeurosis.
- **Insertion**: Lateral side of the base of the fifth proximal phalanx.
- **Function**: Abduction and flexion the little toe.
- **Motor point (MP)**: Proximal one-third point between base of the little toe (A) and heel end (B).

8.6 Flexor hallucis brevis

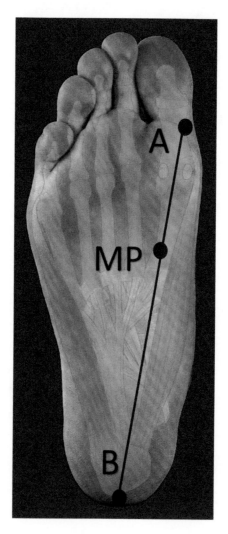

From Moses KP, Nava P, Banks J, Petersen D. Chapter 47 - Foot, Atlas of Clinical Gross Anatomy. 2nd ed.
Elsevier/Saunders; 2013

- **Surface anatomy**: The muscles is one of the deepest foot intrinsic muscles (the third layer) and difficult to be identified superficially.
- **Origin**: Plantar surface of cuboid and cuneiform tarsal bones.
- **Insertion**: Plantar side of the base of the proximal phalanges of the great toe.
- **Function**: Flexion the great toe.
- **Motor point (MP)**[33,34]: Distal one-third point between medial side of the great toe base (A) and heel end (B).
- **Injection tip**: The muscle lies just medial to the adductor halluces oblique head.

8.7 Extensor hallucis brevis

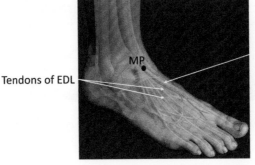

From Moses KP, Nava P, Banks J, Petersen D. Chapter 47 - Foot, Atlas of Clinical Gross Anatomy. 2nd ed. Elsevier/Saunders; 2013

- **Surface anatomy**: superficial muscle covering the lateral dorsum of the foot
- **Origin**: dorsolateral aspect of calcaneus
- **Insertion**: dorsum of the proximal phalanx of the great toe
- **Function**: great toe extension at metatarsophalageal and proximal interphalangeal joints.
- **Motor point (MP)**: At dorsal ankle line, where the extensor hallucis tendon meets the extensor digitorum longus tendon (between the tendons).
- **Injection tip**: Superficial muscle. Isolated great toe extension is seen when the injection needle is located at the MP.

8.8 Extensor digitorum brevis

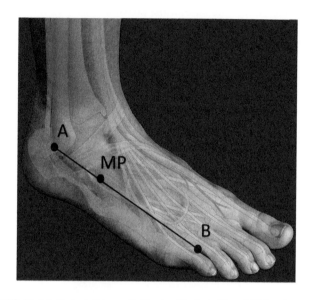

From Moses KP, Nava P, Banks J, Petersen D. Chapter 47 - Foot, Atlas of Clinical Gross Anatomy. 2ⁿᵈ ed.
Elsevier/Saunders; 2013

- **Surface anatomy**: superficial muscle covering the lateral dorsum of the foot
- **Origin**: Dorsolateral aspect of calcaneus
- **Insertion**:dorsum of midphalangeal bones (2–4)
- **Function**: toe extension at metatarsophalageal and proximal interphalangeal joints.
- **Motor point (MP)**: Proximal one-third between lateral malleolus lateral tip (A) and fourth interdigital web (B).
- **Injection tip**: If toes flexion is noted with electrical stimulation, then the need is pulled back (the needle penetrates extensor digitorum brevis).

Motor points injections for deformities

Deformities of head/face/ neck

9.1 Oromandibular dystonia (difficult to open mouth)

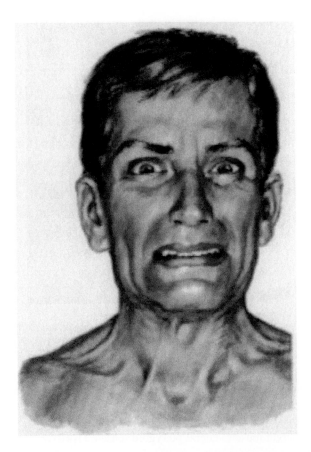

From Werner KM, Ooi WW, McQuillen, DP et al. Chapter 44 - Bacterial Diseases. In: Srinivasan J, Chaves CJ, Scott BJ, Small JE, eds. Netter's Neurology. 3rd ed. Elsevier; 2020

Botulinum Neurotoxin. https://doi.org/10.1016/B978-0-323-69715-6.00015-6

1. Called lockjaw.
2. Clinical feature: reduced mouth opening caused by involuntary spasm of the mastication muscles.
3. Botulinum toxin injection:
   a. Primary target muscles: temporalis (1-1) and masseter (1-2).
   b. Secondary target muscles: medial pterygoid (1-3) only because of technical difficulties.

*In addition, if jaw is deviated to right (left) side, then right (left) lateral pterygoid (1-4) is indicated for injection.

9.2 Oromandibular dystonia (difficult to close mouth)

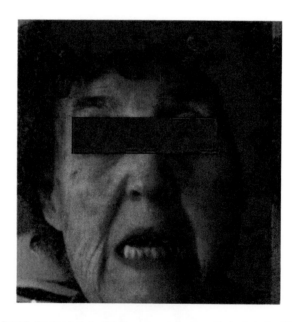

From Teemul TA, Patel R, Kanatas A, Carter LM. Management of oromandibular dystonia with botulinum A toxin: a series of cases. British Journal of Oral and Maxillofacial Surgery. 2016;54(10):1080–1084

1. Clinical feature: difficult to close mouth caused by involuntary spasm of the mouth opening muscles.
2. Botulinum toxin injection:
   a. Primary target muscle: lateral pterygoid muscle (1-4).

9.3 Bruxism (teeth grinding)

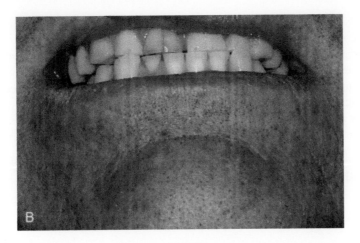

From Allen RP, Salas RE, Gamaldo C. Chapter 11.2 – Movement Disorders in Sleep. In: Kryger MH, ed. Atlas of Clinical Sleep Medicine. 2nd ed. Elsevier/Saunders; 2014

1. Clinical feature: teeth grinding (similar to oromandibular dystonia, difficult to open mouth)
2. Botulinum toxin injection:
   a. Primary target muscles: temporalis (1-1), masseter (1-2), and lateral pterygoid (1-4).
   b. Secondary target muscle: medial pterygoid (1-3) It is recommended as secondary target muscle only because of technical difficulties. If approach to this muscle is not difficult, it could be a primary target muscle.

9.4 Torticollis

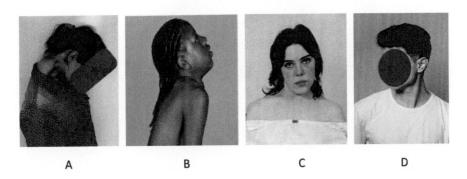

A   B   C   D

(A) From Seliverstov Y, Arestov S, Klyushnikov S, Shpilyukova Y, Illarioshkin S. A methodological approach for botulinum neurotoxin injections to the longus colli muscle in dystonic anterocollis: A case series of 4 patients and a literature review. Journal of Clinical Neuroscience. 2020;80:188–194 ; (B, C) From Herring JA. Chapter 11 - Disorders of the Neck, Tachdjian's Pediatric Orthopaedics. 5th ed. Elsevier/Saunders; 2014

1. Torticollis is classified by the direction of the neck deviation.
2. Target muscles vary with the deviation.
3. Most torticollis is mixed type (combined neck deviations).
4. Well understanding of the muscle function is very important to select target muscles.
5. Motor points depend on type of torticollis.

9.5 Anterocollis

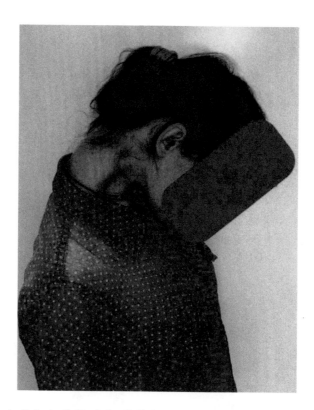

From Seliverstov Y, Arestov S, Klyushnikov S, Shpilyukova Y, Illarioshkin S. A methodological approach for botulinum neurotoxin injections to the longus colli muscle in dystonic anterocollis: A case series of 4 patients and a literature review. Journal of Clinical Neuroscience. 2020;80:188–194.

1. Clinical feature: difficult to extend neck caused by involuntary contraction of the neck flexor muscles.
2. Botulinum toxin injection:
   Target muscle: bilateral sternocleidomastoid (1-15), platysma (1-11), longus capitis (1-16), and longus collis (1-17). Because of deep location, ultrasound is recommended to localize longus capitis and collis.

9.6 **Retrocollis**

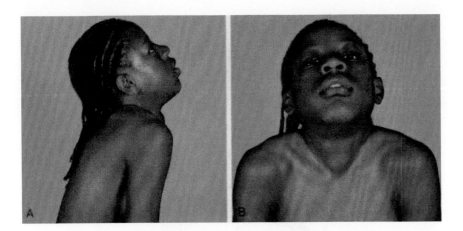

From Herring JA. Chapter 11 - Disorders of the Neck, Tachdjian's Pediatric Orthopaedics. 5th ed. Elsevier/Saunders; 2014

1. Clinical feature: difficult to flex neck caused by involuntary contraction of the neck extensor muscles.
2. Botulinum toxin injection:
   Target muscles: semispinalis capitis and cervicis (1-5 & 1-6), splenius capitis and cervicis (1-7 & 1-8), longissimus capitis and cervicis (1-9 & 1-10), and upper trapezius (1-19).

9.7 Laterocollis

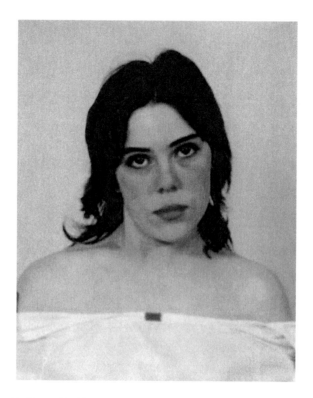

From Herring JA. Chapter 11 - Disorders of the Neck, Tachdjian's Pediatric Orthopaedics. 5th ed. Elsevier/ Saunders; 2014

1. Clinical feature: difficult to keep neck vertical caused by involuntary contraction of the neck ipsilateral lateral flexor muscles.
2. Botulinum toxin injection:
   Target muscles: ipsilateral scalene muscles (1-11, 11-12, & 11-13), sternocleidomastoid (1-15), levator scapulae (1-18), and upper trapezius (1-19).

9.8 **Rotatocollis**

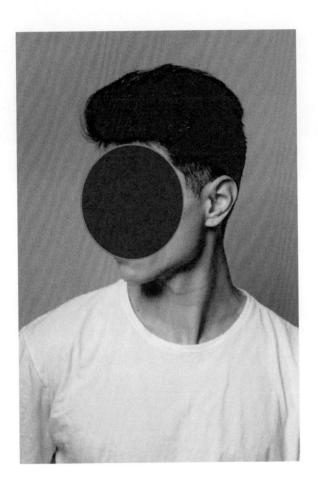

1. Clinical feature: Twisted neck caused by involuntary contraction of the neck rotator muscles.
2. Botulinum toxin injection:
   Target muscles: ipsilateral splenius capitis and cervicis (1-7 & 1-8), contralateral sternocleidomastoid (1-15).

9.9 Shoulder elevation

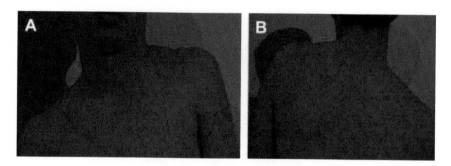

From Jankovic J. Peripherally induced movement disorders. Neurologic Clinics. 2009;27(3):821–832.

1. Clinical feature: Shrugged shoulder(s). May combined with torticollis. In the picture, the left shoulder is elevated (A, anterior and B, posterior)
2. Botulinum toxin injection:
   Target muscles: ipsilateral levator scapulae (1-18), upper trapezius (1-19), and scalen muscles (1-12 to 1-14).
   If torticollis is combined, target muscles are selected based on type of torticollis (see 9-5 to 9-8)

Deformities of trunk

10.1 Opisthotonos

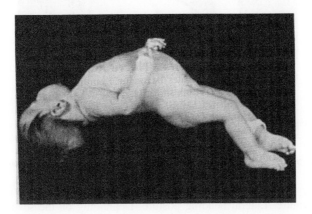

From Kliegman RM, St Geme JW 3rd. Nelson Textbook of Pediatrics. 21ˢᵗ ed. Elsevier; 2020: p. 3058

1. Clinical feature: whole spinal extension posture. Depending on the severity of spine extension level, back extensor muscles are targeted.
2. Botulinum toxin injection: bilaterally. Target muscles at each spinal level.
   a. Cervical level extensors: semispinalis capitis and cervicis (1-5 & 1-6), splenius capitis and cervicis (1-7 & 1-8), and longissimus capitis and cervicis (1-9 & 1-10).
   b. Thoracic level extensors: several parathoracic spinal extensors (2-2)
   c. Lumbar level extensors: several paralumbar spinal extensors (2-2).

Botulinum Neurotoxin. https://doi.org/10.1016/B978-0-323-69715-6.00007-7

10.2 **Scoliosis**

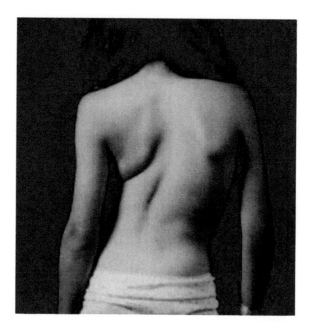

From Herring JA. Chapter 12 - Scoliosis, Tachdjian's Pediatric Orthopaedics. 5th ed. Elsevier/Saunders; 2014

1. Clinical feature: Lateral bending posture. Depending on the severity of spinal bending level, bulged paraspinal muscles (concave side) targeted.
2. Botulinum toxin injection: unilaterally (concave side) at every 2-3 vertebral levels.
   a. Cervical level paraspinal muscles (concave side) and lateral flexors (see 9-7).
   b. Thoracic level paraspinal muscles (concave side) (2-2)
   c. Lumbar level paraspinal muscles (concave side) (2-2).

Deformities of upper arm

11

11.1 Decerebrate rigidity (upper arm level)

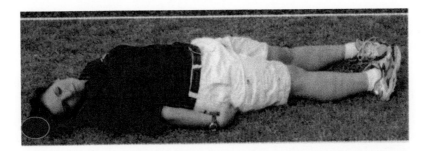

From Magee DJ. Chapter 2 - Head and Face, Orthopedic Physical Assessment. 6th ed. Elsevier/Saunders; 2014

1. Clinical feature: shoulder adduction-extension-internal rotation and elbow extension posture on supine.
2. Botulinum toxin injection:
   a. Primary target muscles:
   shoulder adductors: pectoralis major (3-1), corachobrachialis (3-2), latissimus dorsi (3-3).
   shoulder internal rotators: pectoralis major (3-1), latissimus dorsi (3-3), subscapularis (3-6), teres major (3-10).
   b. Secondary target muscles:
   shoulder extensors: posterior deltoid (3-12), triceps long head (3-14).

Botulinum Neurotoxin. https://doi.org/10.1016/B978-0-323-69715-6.00013-2

11.2 Decorticate rigidity (upper arm level)

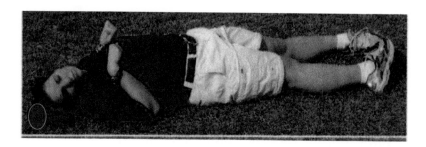

From Magee DJ. Chapter 2 - Head and Face, Orthopedic Physical Assessment. 6th ed. Elsevier/Saunders; 2014

1. Clinical feature: shoulder adduction-internal rotation and elbow flexion posture on supine.
2. Botulinum toxin injection:
   Primary target muscles:
   shoulder adductors/internal rotators: pectoralis major (3-1), corachobrachialis (3-2), latissimus dorsi (3-3), subscapularis (3-6), teres major (3-10).

11.3 Tonic labyrinth posture at supine

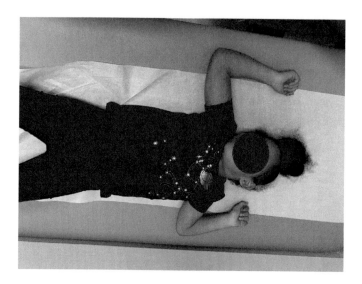

1. Clinical feature: scapular retraction, shoulder external rotation-abduction and elbow flexion bilaterally on supine.
2. Botulinum toxin injection:
   a. Primary target muscles:
   shoulder external rotators: infraspinatus (3-5), teres minor (3-11), posterior deltoid (3-12).
   scapular retractors: middle trapezius (1-17), rhomboid major & minor (3-7 & 3-8).
   b. Secondary target muscles:
   shoulder abductors: supraspinatus (3-4) and middle deltoid (3-12).

11.4 **Hemiplegic arm (upper arm level)**

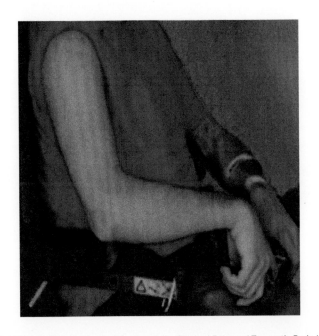

From Kozin SH, Lightdale-Miric N. Chapter 32 - Spasticity: Cerebral Palsy and Traumatic Brain Injury. In: Wolfe SW, Pederson WC, Kozin SH, Cohen MS, eds. Green's Operative Hand Surgery. 7th ed. Elsevier; 2017

1. Clinical feature: shoulder adduction-internal rotation and elbow flexion (see 12-3 for forearm and hand deformities of hemiplegic arm). It is becoming more pronounced while walking.
2. Botulinum toxin injection:
   a. Primary target muscles:
   Shoulder adductors (3-1, 3-2, & 3-3) and internal rotators (3-1, 3-3, 3-6, & 3-7).
   Elbow flexors (3-15).

b. Secondary target muscles:
Other elbow flexors, biceps brachii (3-13) and brachialis (4-1) can be indicated for severe elbow flexor hypertonia.

Note: Three elbow flexors (brachialis, biceps brachii, and brachioradialis) have different roles in elbow flexion depending on forearm position (see injection notes of 3-13, 3-15, & 4-1).

CHAPTER

Deformities of forearm 12

12.1 Decerebrate rigidity (forearm level)

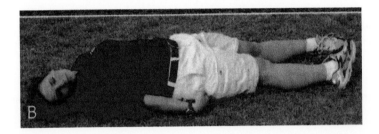

From Magee DJ. Chapter 2 - Head and Face, Orthopedic Physical Assessment. 6th ed. Elsevier/Saunders; 2014

1. Clinical feature: elbow extension and forearm pronated posture on supine.
2. Botulinum toxin injection:
   Primary target muscles: triceps (3-14) and pronator teres (4-2)

   Note: pronator quadratus is more active pronator at elbow flexion position (pronator teres is active at elbow extension).

Botulinum Neurotoxin. https://doi.org/10.1016/B978-0-323-69715-6.00012-0

12.2 Decorticate rigidity (forearm level)

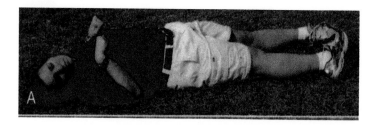

From Magee DJ. Chapter 2 - Head and Face, Orthopedic Physical Assessment. 6th ed. Elsevier/Saunders; 2014

1. Clinical feature: elbow flexion posture with forearm supination or pronation on supine.
2. Botulinum toxin injection:
   a. Primary target muscles: elbow flexors (see note below): biceps brachii (3-13), brachialis (3-15), brachioradialis (4-1).
   b. Secondary target muscles: depending on forearm position (supinated or pronated).

Note: biceps brachii is a major elbow flexor at the forearm supinated, brachialis at the forearm pronated, and brachiodradialis at the forearm neutral position.

12.3 Hemiplegic arm (forearm level)

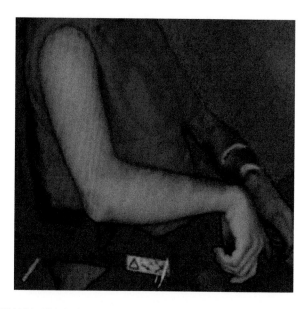

From Kozin SH, Lightdale-Miric N. Chapter 32 - Spasticity: Cerebral Palsy and Traumatic Brain Injury. In: Wolfe SW, Pederson WC, Kozin SH, Cohen MS, eds. Green's Operative Hand Surgery. 7th ed. Elsevier; 2017

1. Clinical feature: Forearm pronation (more common than forearm supination), wrist flexion (with radial or ulnar deviation), and finger flexion posture. It is becoming more pronounced while walking.
2. Botulinum toxin injection:
   Primary target muscles: pronator teres (4-2) and quadratus (4-3) if the forearm pronated. Wrist flexors, depending on radial or ulnar deviation, (4-4, 4-5, & 4-6). Thumb opponens (5-2), flexors (4-9 & 5-3), adductors (5-4). Finger flexors: flexor digitorum superficialis and profundus (4-7 & 8).

Note: If the forearm is supinated (Figure in "12.2 Decorticate rigicdity (foream level)"), biceps brachii (3-13) and supinator (4-18) are to be targeted instead of brachialis.

Deformities of hand

13.1 Wrist drop

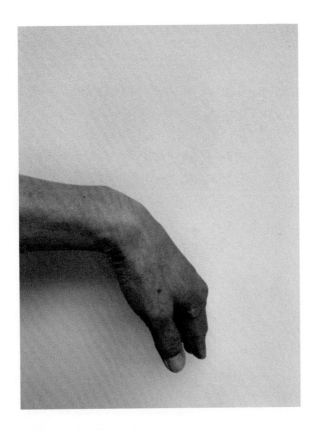

1. Clinical feature: wrist flexion with/without ulnar or radial deviation.
2. Botulinum toxin injection:

    a. Primary target muscles: wrist flexors: palmaris longus (4-4), flexor carpi radialis and/or ulnaris (4-5 & 4-6) depending on deviation (radial or ulnar).

    b. Secondary target muscles: finger flexors: flexor digitorum superficialis & profundus (4-7 & 8), only if finger flexors hypertonia is combined.

13.2 Cortical thumb

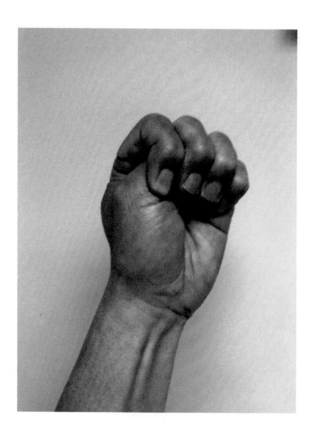

1. Clinical feature: clenched fist but thumb is covered by other four fingers.

2. Botulinum toxin injection:

    a. Primary target muscles: thumb opponens (5-2), adductor (5-4), and flexors (4-9 & 5-3, see note) finger flexors: flexor digitourm superficialis & profundus (4-7 & 8).

Note: If thumb interphalangeal joint is not flexed, flexor pollicis longus is not targeted.

13.3 Hand intrinsic minus (claw hand)

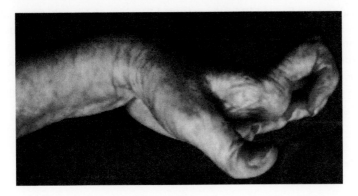

From Kozin SH, Lightdale-Miric N. Chapter 32 - Spasticity: Cerebral Palsy and Traumatic Brain Injury. In: Wolfe SW, Pederson WC, Kozin SH, Cohen MS, eds. Green's Operative Hand Surgery. 7th ed. Elsevier; 2017

1. Clinical feature: Primarily metacarpophalangeal joints hyperextended secondarily interphalangeal joints flexed due to imbalance between strong hand extrinsic and weak hand intrinsic muscles.
2. Botulinum toxin injection:
   a. Primary target muscles: external finger extensors: extensor digitourm communis (4-13)
   b. Secondary target muscles: wrist extensors: extensor carpi radialis (4-10 & 4-11) and/or ulnaris (4-12). Finger flexors: flexor digitourm superficialis & profundus (4-7 & 8).

13.4 Hand intrinsic plus

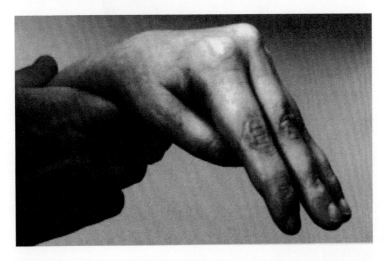

From Kozin SH, Lightdale-Miric N. Chapter 32 - Spasticity: Cerebral Palsy and Traumatic Brain Injury. In: Wolfe SW, Pederson WC, Kozin SH, Cohen MS, eds. Green's Operative Hand Surgery. 7th ed. Elsevier; 2017

1. Clinical feature: flexed MP joints, extended IP joints, and mostly finger adducted due to imbalance between strong hand intrinsic and weak extrinsic muscles.
2. Botulinum toxin injection:
   a. Primary target muscles: hand intrinsic muscles: lumbricals (5-7) & palmar interossei (5-10).
   b. Secondary target muscle: extensor indicis (4-17): especially for the index finger.

13.5 Trigger finger(s)

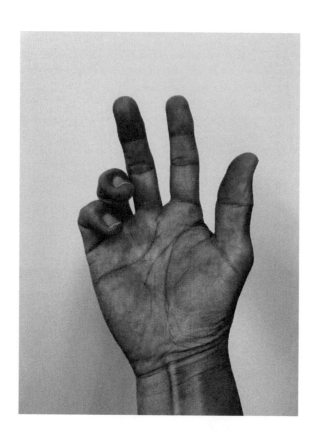

1. Clinical feature: finger flexed at IP joints. Target muscles are selected depending on affected fingers.
2. Botulinum toxin injection:
   Primary target muscles:
   for thumb trigger: flexor pollicis longus (4-9)
   for 2nd to 4th trigger: flexor digitorum superficialis & profundus (4-7 & 4-8).

Deformities of upper leg

14.1 Wind swept leg

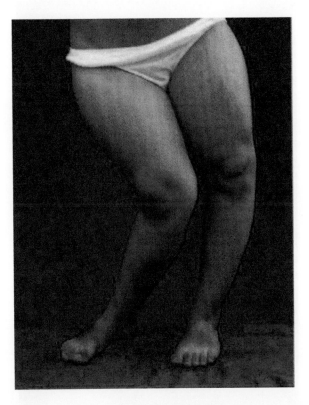

From Kocaoglu M, Bilen FE. Fixator-assisted nailing for correction of long bone deformities. Operative Techniques in Orthopaedics. 2011;21(2):163–173

1. Clinical feature: One hip (right at the picture) flexed-internally rotated-adducted and the other one (left at the picture) flexed-externally rotated-abducted and bilateral knee flexed.

Botulinum Neurotoxin. https://doi.org/10.1016/B978-0-323-69715-6.00017-X

2. Botulinum toxin injection: different target muscles depending on hip side (at the picture the hip is windswept to the left)
   a. Target muscles for internally rotated-adducted hip (right hip at the picture): iliopsoas (6-1), tensor fascia lata (6-2), hip adductors (6-9 to 6-12), hamstrings (6-17 & 18)
   b. Target muscles for externally rotated-abducted hip (left hip at the picture): iliopsoas (6-1), hamstrings (6-17 & 18) if hip flexion and knee flexion deformities are combined.

14.2 **Knocked knee**

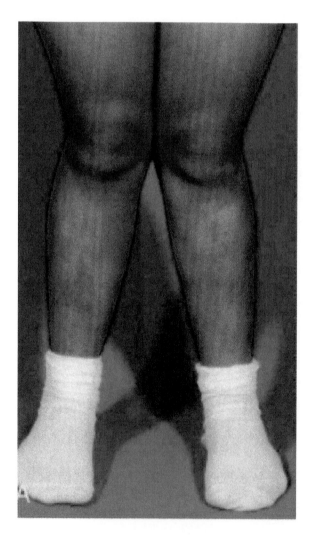

From Herring JA. Chapter 22 - Disorders of the Leg, Tachdjian's Pediatric Orthopaedics. 5th ed. Elsevier/
Saunders; 2014

1. Clinical feature: Each knee crosses midline with hip adduction. More pronounced while standing and walking. Pes planovalgus deformity is usually combined.
2. Botulinum toxin injection:
   a. Primary target muscles: hip adductors (6-9 to 6-12)
   b. Secondary target muscles: tensor fascia lata (6-2) and peroneus muscles (7-4 to 7-6) depending on how severely the hip is internal rotated and foot pronated.

14.3 Crouching

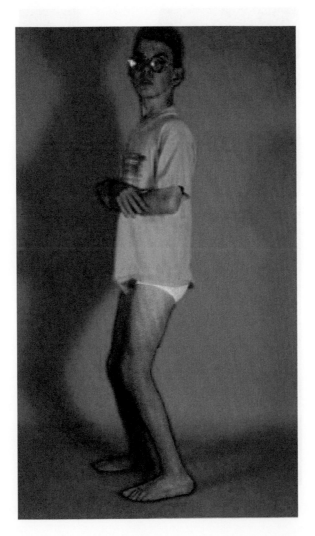

From Herring JA. Chapter 35 - Disorders of the Brain, Tachdjian's Pediatric Orthopaedics. 5th ed. Elsevier/ Saunders; 2014

1. Clinical feature: Unable to extend knees while standing and walking.
2. Botulinum toxin injection:
   a. Primary target muscles: hamstrings (6-17 & 18)
   b. Secondary target muscles: gastrocnemius (7-1 & 2).

14.4 Hyperextended knee (genu recurvatum)

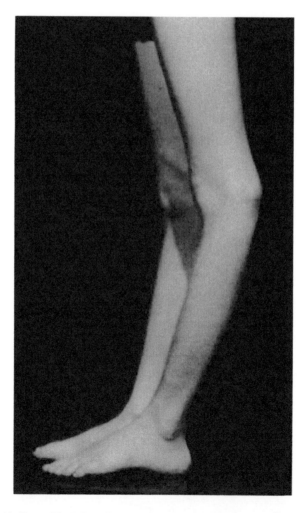

From Herring JA. Chapter 37 - Poliomyelitis, Tachdjian's Pediatric Orthopaedics. 5ᵗʰ ed. Elsevier/Saunders;
2014

1. Clinical feature: Excessive knee hyperextension. More pronounced at standing or supine position (decerebrate or decorticate rigidity).
2. Botulinum toxin injection:
   a. Primary target muscles: knee extensors (6-13 to 6-16).

14.5 Hemiplegic leg (upper leg level)

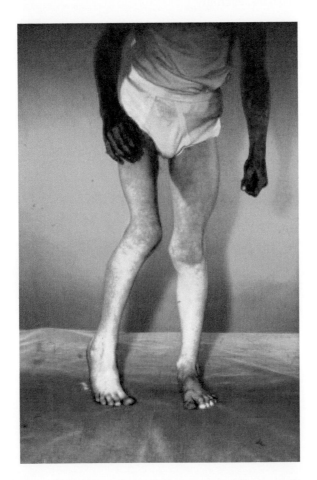

From Tsirikos AI, Eunson P. Chapter 26 - The paediatric spine and neuromuscular conditions. In: Luqmani R, Robb J, Porter D, Joseph B, eds. Textbook of Orthopaedics, Trauma, and Rheumatology. 2nd ed. Elsevier/Mosby Ltd.; 2013

1. Clinical feature (right hemiplegic leg at the picture): stereotype of hip internal rotation, lack of knee flexion, plantar flexion, and inversion (at the picture) or eversion at standing. Pronounced while walking.
3. Botulinum toxin injection:
   a. Primary target muscles: tensor fascia lata (6-2)
   b. Secondary target muscles: quadriceps (6-13 to 6-16): in case of knee flexion deficiency during swing phase. Injection to rectus femoris can cause week hip flexion at initial swing. Hamstrings (6-17 & 6-18): in case of crouching or severe equinus deformity.

Deformities of lower leg

15

15.1 Hemiplegic leg (lower leg level)

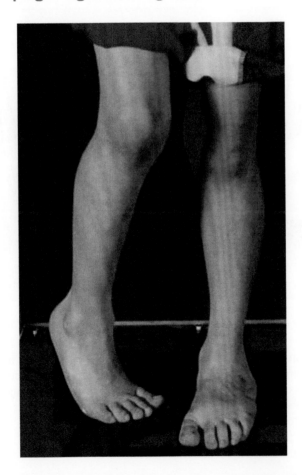

From Herring JA. Chapter 35 - Disorders of the Brain, Tachdjian's Pediatric Orthopaedics. 5th ed. Elsevier/
Saunders; 2014

Botulinum Neurotoxin. https://doi.org/10.1016/B978-0-323-69715-6.00018-1

1. Clinical feature (right hemiplegic leg at the picture): stereotype of hip internal rotation, lack of knee flexion, plantar flexion, and foot inversion (at the picture) or eversion, and toe flexion at standing. Pronounced while standing and walking.
2. Botulinum toxin injection:
   a. Primary target muscles: gastrocnemius (7-1 & 2), soleus (7-3)
   b. Secondary target muscles:
      tibialis posterior (7-8): in case of foot inversion.
      peroneus (7-4 to 7-6): in case of foot eversion
      flexor digitorum longus 7-11) & brevis (8-4): in case of significant toe flexions

15.2 In-toeing

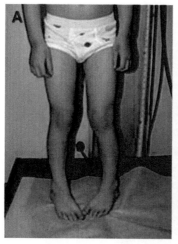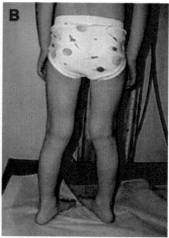

From Harris E. The intoeing child. Clinics in Podiatric Medicine and Surgery. 2013;30(4):531–565.

1. Clinical feature: toes turn inward commonly combined with foot inversion. It is resulted from pelvic anteversion, tibial torsion, or forefoot adduction (see 16. Deformities of foot). Depending on the level of abnormality, the injection target muscles are selected.
2. Botulinum toxin injection:
   a. Primary target muscles:
      tibialis posterior (7- 8), abductor hallucis (8-1)

b. Secondary target muscles:
tibialis anterior (7-7): if foot inversion is so severe (tibialis anterior is a strong foot invertor).
tensor fascia lata (6-2): in case of hip internal rotation is present
gastrocnemius and soleus (7-1 to 7-3): in case of plantar flexion combined.

15.3 **Out-toeing**

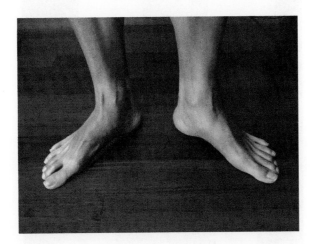

1. Clinical feature: toes turn outward commonly combined with pes valgus and flat foot. It is resulted from physiologic development (infantile hip joint contracture), pelvic retroversion, and tibial external torsion.
2. Botulinum toxin injection:
   a. Primary target muscles:
   peroneus muscles (7- 4 to 7-6)
   b. Secondary target muscles:
   gastrocnemius and soleus (7-1 to 7-3): in case of equinus combined.
   gluteus maximus (6-3) and hip extensors (6-6): in case of externally rotated hip.

15.4 **Pes equinus**

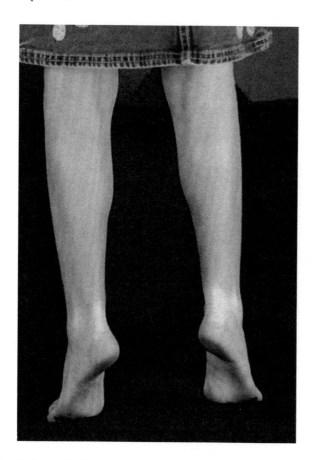

*From Herring JA. Chapter 23 - Disorders of the Foot, Tachdjian's Pediatric Orthopaedics. 5ᵗʰ ed. Elsevier/
Saunders; 2014*

1. Clinical features: limited ankle dorsiflexion deformity. Standing with forefoot/ toe weight bearing. If ankle dorsiflexion is limited at both knee flexion and extension position, both gastrocnemius and soleus muscles are tight. If ankle dorsiflexion is limited only at knee extension position, gastrocnemius muscle is tight.

2. Botulinum toxin injection:
   a. Primary target muscles:
      gastrocnemius muscle (7-1 & 2), soleus (7-3): If ankle dorsiflexion limitation is significantly different between knee flexion and extension position (see clinical feature), it is advised to inject more botulinum toxins to the gastrocnemius than soleus.

b. Secondary target muscles:
   tibialis posterior (7-8): in case of foot inversion is combined.
   peroneus longus and brevis (7-4 & 5): in case of foot eversion is combined.
   flexor digitorum longus (7-11): in case of toe flexion deformity is combined.

15.5 Equinovarus

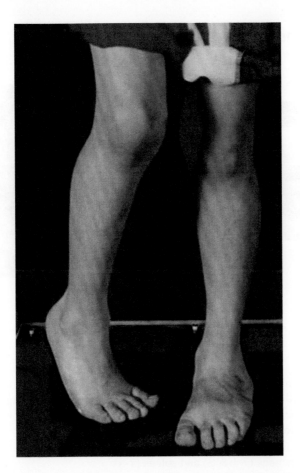

From Herring JA. Chapter 35 - Disorders of the Brain, Tachdjian's Pediatric Orthopaedics. 5th ed. Elsevier/
Saunders; 2014

1. Clinical feature: Deformity of foot with limited ankle dorsiflexion and toes inward turning. Standing with weight bearing along the lateral border of the midfoot/forefoot.

2. Botulinum toxin injection:
   a. Primary target muscles:
      gastrocnemius (7-1 & 2) and soleus (7-3)
      tibialis posterior (7-8)
   b. Secondary target muscles:
      tibialis anterior (7-7): tibialis anterior is another strong foot invertor.
      abductor hallucis (8-1).
      flexor digitorum longus (7-11): in case of toe flexion combined.

15.6 Equinovalgus

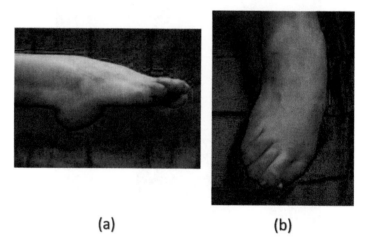

(a)   (b)

From Myerson MS, Ferrao PN, Clowers BE. Management of paralytic equinovalgus deformity. Foot and Ankle Clinics. 2011;16(3):489–497.

1. Clinical feature: Deformity of foot with limited ankle dorsiflexion (Fig. a) and toes outward turning (Fig. b). Standing with weight bearing along the medial border of the forefoot.
2. Botulinum toxin injection:
   a. Primary target muscles:
      Gastrocnemius (7-1 & 2) and soleus (7-3)
      Peroneus muscles (7-4 to 7-6).
   b. Secondary target muscles:
      flexor digitorum longus (7-11): in case of toe flexion combined.

Deformities of foot

16

16.1 Hallux valgus

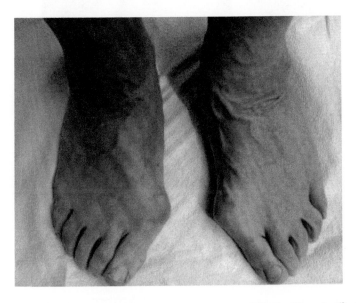

From Swartz MH. Chapter 20 - The Musculoskeletal System, Textbook of Physical Diagnosis. 8th ed. Elsevier; 2020

1. Clinical feature: Great toe deviates laterally (left foot in the picture). Usually combined with overriding toe deformity and pronated foot.
2. Botulinum toxin injection:
   a. Primary target muscles: adductor hallucis transverse (8-2) and oblique (8-3).
   b. Secondary target muscles: peroneus muscles (7-4 to 7-6) in case of foot pronation combined.

Botulinum Neurotoxin. https://doi.org/10.1016/B978-0-323-69715-6.00019-3

16.2 Hallux varus

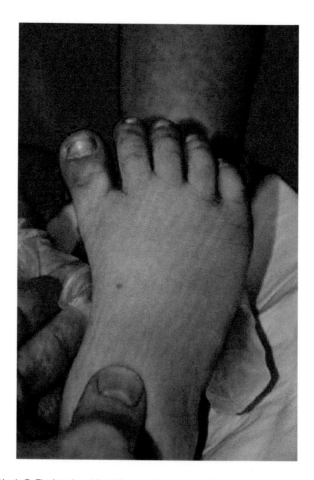

From Harris E. The intoeing child. Clinics in Podiatric Medicine and Surgery. 2013;30(4):531–565.

1. Clinical feature: Great toe deviates medially (in-toeing). Usually combined with overriding toe deformity and pronated foot.
2. Botulinum toxin injection:
   a. Primary target muscles: abductor hallucis (8-1)
   b. Secondary target muscles: tibialis posterior and/or anterior in case of foot supination combined.

16.3 **Claw toes**

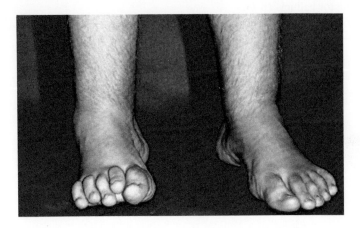

From Deeney VF, Arnold J. Chapter 22 — Orthopedics. In: Zitelli B, McIntire S, Nowalk A, eds. Zitelli and Davis'
Atlas of Pediatric Physical Diagnosis. 7th ed. Elsevier; 2018

1. Clinical feature: Limited toe extension deformity.
2. Botulinum toxin injection:
   a. Primary target muscles: flexor digitorum longus (7-11) and brevis (8-4): for toes except great toe. Flexor hallucis long (7-12) and brevis (8-6): for great toe.

16.4 **Forefoot adduction (metatarsus adductus)**

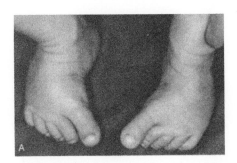
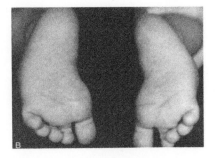

From Herring JA. Chapter 23 - Disorders of the Foot, Tachdjian's Pediatric Orthopaedics. 5th ed. Elsevier/
Saunders; 2014

3. Clinical feature: Forefoot is twisted medially (in-toeing).
4. Botulinum toxin injection:
   a. Primary target muscles: Tibialis anterior and posterior (7-7 & 7-8) and abductor hallucis (8-1).
   Note: tibialis anterior is an ankle dorsiflexor, but also a strong foot inverter.

Appendix: Salivary and sweat glands

A. Injections to the salivary glands for drooling
A.1 Parotid gland

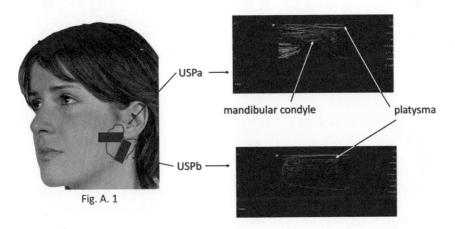

USPa →

mandibular condyle   platysma

USPb →

Fig. A. 1

From Logan BM, Reynolds PA, Rice S, Hutchings R. McMinn's Color Atlas of Head and Neck Anatomy. 5th ed.
Elsevier; 2017

- **Surface anatomy:** Superficial organ just under the skin at the face and platysma muscle at neck. The largest gland is located anterior, posterior, inferior to the low ear lobe (mastoid is posterior, zygomatic arch is anterior, and mandibular angle is inferior margin) (Fig. A.1, Left parotid gland heart shape in red color and ultrasound probe a (USPa) and b (USPb).
- **Function:** Activated when smells or chews food. Less active in resting state. Major component is serous secretion.
- **Injection point:** Any point in the gland.
- **Injection tip:** Ultrasound helps to localize the gland and injection needle. Salivary glands are more hyperechogenic than muscle (lighter than muscle). Upper and lower ultrasound images are obtained when ultrasound probe is applied horizontally (USPa) and vertically (USPb). Bigger images can be obtained with vertical application of ultrasound probe between the mandibular ramus and sternocleidomastoid muscle. Injections may be divided into several sites.

A.2 Submandibular (submaxillary) gland

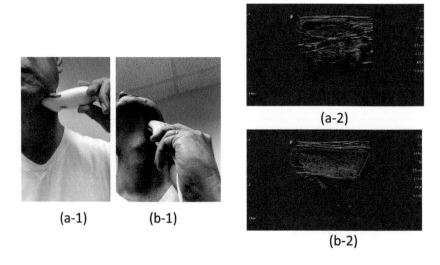

(a-1)   (b-1)

(a-2)

(b-2)

- **Surface anatomy:** Superficial organ just under the platysma muscle at outside of floor of mouth. The gland is located anteromedial to the mandibular angle (mid-point between the mandibular angle and chin).
- **Function:** Majorly active in resting state and becomes less active when smells or chews food (parotid glands become major active gland). Major component is mixed with serous and mucous secretion.
- **Injection point:** Any point in the gland.
- **Injection tip:** Ultrasound helps to localize the gland and injection needle. Salivary glands are more hyperechogenic than muscle (lighter than muscle). Because the gland is protected by the mandible laterally, it is very critical to maintain neck hyperextension positioning and to approach caudo-cephalic direction for successful injections (please note the angles of the ultrasound probes in figure a-1 and b-1 and corresponding ultrasound images in a-2 and b-2; submandibular glands are marked in red). Bigger images can be obtained with neck hyperextension (b-2). Injections may be divided into several sites.

A.3 Sublingual gland

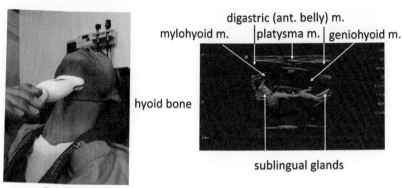

Fig. A.3

- **Surface anatomy:** Deep organ under the tongue (between tongue and mouth floor muscles). Unable to be seen by naked eyes. The gland is the smallest major salivary gland and is located inferolateral to the tongue.
- **Function:** Major component is mucous secretion.
- **Injection point:** Any point in the gland.
- **Injection tip:** Because of high vasculature of the mouth floor, there is a high risk of bleeding with injection. Salivary glands are more hyperechogenic than muscle (lighter than muscle). Neck hyperextension is needed for this procedure (Fig. A.3). Ultrasound helps to localize the gland and injection needle (see ultrasound image).

B. Injections to the sweat glands for hyperhidrosis

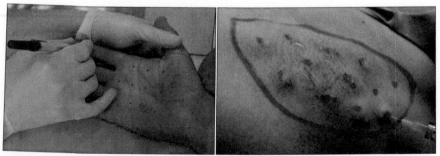

Fig. B.1   Fig. B.2

(B.1) *From Mariwalla K, Solish N. Chapter 27 - Palmoplantar Hyperhidrosis. In: Carruthers A, Carruthers J, eds. Botulinum Toxin - Procedures in Cosmetic Dermatology Series. 4th ed. Elsevier; 2018; (B.2) From Glaser DA, Mattox AR. Chapter 26 - Focal Axillary Hyperhidrosis. In: Carruthers A, Carruthers J, eds. Botulinum Toxin - Procedures in Cosmetic Dermatology Series. 4th ed. Elsevier; 2018*

- **Surface anatomy:** All sweat glands are under the skin (in dermal layer). Densely located in palms, soles, axillar, and pubic areas.
- **Function:** Body temperature regulation.
- **Injection point:** Multiple injection points.
- **Injection tip:** Multiple intradermal injections are most effective. Distance between injections 1−2 cm is recommended (see Fig. B.1 & B.2). Multiple injections to the palms or soles are painful. Cold spray or local topical anesthetics (lidocaine cream) are helpful to decrease the injection pain. The outcome of the injections can be noticed earlier than muscle injections.

Bibliography

Head/face/neck

1. Schwartz M, Freund B. Treatment of temporomandibular disorders with botulinum toxin. *Clin J Pain*. 2002;18(6, Supp):S198–S203.
2. Chang Y, Cantelmi D, Wisco JJ, Fattah A, Hannam AG, Agur AM. Evidence for the functional compartmentalization of the temporalis muscle: a 3-dimensional study of innervation. *J Oral Maxillofac Surg*. 2013;71(7):1170–1177.
3. Carillo RJC. Pterygoid botulinum toxin injection. *Philipp J Otolaryngol Head Neck Surg*. 2011;26(1):55–56.
4. Yoshida K. Computer-aided design/computer-assisted manufacture-derived needle guide for injection of botulinum toxin into the lateral pterygoid muscle in patients with oromandibular dystonia. *J Oral Facial Pain Headache*. 2018;32:e13–e21.
5. Trindade de Almeida, Carruthers J. In: Carruthers J, Carruthers A, eds. *Platysma, Nefertiti Lift, and Beyond; Botulinum Toxin: Procedures in Cosmetic Dermatology Series, Chapter 22*. 4th ed. Edinburgh: Elsevier; 2018:145–151.
6. Falla D, Dall'Alba P, Rainoldi A, Merletti R, Jull G. Location of innervation zones of sternocleidomastoid and scalene muscles-a basis for clinical and research electromyography applications. *Clin Neurophysiol*. 2002;113:57–63.
7. Delnooz CCCS, Venugen LC, Pasman JW, Lapatki BG, van Dijk JP, van de Warrenburg BPC. The clinical utility of botulinum toxin injections targeted at the motor endplate zone in cervical dystonia. *Eur J Neurol*. 2014;21:1486–1492.
8. Seliverstov Y, Arestov S, Klyushnikov S, Shpilyukova Y, Illarioshkin S. A methodological approach for botulinum neurotoxin injections to the longus colli muscle in dystonic anterocollis: a case series of 4 patients and a literature review. *J Clin Neurosci*. 2020;80:188–194.

Trunk

9. Franz A, Klaas J, Schumann M, Frankewitsch T, Filler TJ, Behringer M. Anatomical versus functional motor points of selected upper body muscles. *Muscle Nerve*. 2018;57(3):460–465.
10. Behringer M, Franz Λ, McCourt M, Mester J. Motor point map of upper body muscles. *Eur J Appl Physiol*. 2014;114:1605–1617.

Upper arm

11. Harrison TP, Sadnicka A, Eastwood DM. Motor points for the neuromuscular blockade of the subscapularis muscle. *Arch Phys Med Rehabil*. 2007;88:295–297.
12. Unlu E, Sen T, Esmer AF, Tuccar E, Elhan A, Cakci A. A new technique for subscapularis muscle needle insertion. *Am J Phys Med Rehabil*. 2008;87:710–713.

Forearm

13. Liu J, Pho RWH, Pereira BP, Lau H-K, Kumar VP. Distribution of primary motor motor nerve braches and terminal nerve entry points to the forearm muscles. *Anat Rec.* 1997; 248:456—463.
14. Roberts C, Crystal R, Eastwood DM. Optimal injection points for the neuromuscular blockade of forearm flexor muscles: a cadaveric study. *J Pediatr Orthop.* 2006;15: 351—355.

Hand

15. Im S, Han SH, Choi JH, et al. Anatomic localization of motor points for the neuromuscular blockade of hand intrinsic muscles involved in thumb-in-palm. *Am J Phys Med Rehabil.* 2008;87(9):703—709.

Upper leg

16. Willenborg MJ, Shilt JS, Smith BP, Estrada RL, Castle JA, Koman LA. Technique for iliopsoas ultrasound-guided active electromyography-directed botulinum A toxin injection in cerebral palsy. *J Pediatr Orthop.* 2002;22(2):165—168.
17. Van Campenhout A, Molenaers G. Localization of the motor endplate zone in huma skeletal muscles of the lower limb: anatomical guidelines for injection with botulinum toxin. *Dev Med Child Neurol.* 2011;53:108—119.
18. Van Campenhout A, Verhaegen A, Pans S, Molenaers G. Botulinum toxin type A injections in the psoas muscle of children with cerebral palsy: muscle atrophy after motor end plate-targeted injections. *Res Dev Disabil.* 2013;34:1052—1058.
19. Westhoff B, Seller K, Wild A, Jaeger M, Krauspe R. Ultrasound-guided botulinum toxin injection technique for the iliopsoas muscle. *Dev Med Child Neurol.* 2003;45(12): 829—832.
20. Garcia Ruiz PJ, Perez Higueras A, Quinones D, Escorihuela R, Castillo F. Posterior CT guided approach for botulinum toxin injection into spinal psoas. *J Neurol.* 2003;250(5): 617—618.
21. Crystal RC, Malone AA, Eastwood DM. Motor points for neuromuscular blockade of the adductor muscle group. *Clin Orthop Relat Res.* 2005;437:196—200.
22. Van Campenhout A, Bar-On L, Desloovere K, Huenaerts C, Molenaers G. Motor endplate-targeted botulinum toxin injections of the gracilis muscle in children with cerebral palsy. *Dev Med Child Neurol.* 2015;57(5):476—483.
23. Botter A, Oprandi G, Lanfranco F, Allasia S, Maffiuletti NA, Minetto MA. Atlas of the muscle motor points for the lower limb: implications for electrical stimulation procedres and electrode positioning. *Eur J Appl Physiol.* 2011;111:2461—2471.
24. Albert T, Yelnik A, Colle F, Bonan I, Lassau JP. Anatomic motor point localization for partial quadriceps block in spasticity. *Arch Phys Med Rehabil.* 2000;81(3):285—287.
25. Weiss A, Glaviano NR, Resch J, Saliba S. Reliability of a novel approach for quadriceps motor point assessment. *Muscle Nerve.* 2018;57(1):E1—E7.
26. Rha DW, Yi KH, Park ES, Park C, Kim HJ. Intramuscular nerve distribution of the hamstring muscles: Application to treating spasticity. *Clin Anat.* 2016;29(6):746—751.

Lower leg

27. Hefter H, Nickels W, Samadzadeh S, Rosenthal D. Comparing soleus injections and gastrocnemius injections of botulinum toxin for treating adult spastic foot drop: a monocentric observational study. *J Int Med Res.* 2021;49(3):1—13.

28. Sheverdin VA, Hur MS, Won SY, Song WC, Hu KS, Koh KS. Extra-and intramuscular nerves distributions of the triceps surae muscle as a basis for muscle resection and botulinum toxin injections. *Surg Radiol Anat.* 2009;31:615—621.

29. Parratte B, Tatu L, Vuillier F, Diop M, Monnier G. Intramuscular distribution of nerves in the human triceps surae muscle: anatomical bases for treatment of spastic drop foot with botulinum toxin. *Surg Radiol Anat.* 2002;24:91—96.

30. Lee JH, Lee BN, An X, Chung RH, Han SH. Location of the motor entry point and intramuscular motor point of the tibialis posterior muscle: for effective motor point block. *Clin Anat.* 2011;24(1):91—96.

31. Yi K-H, Rha D-W, Lee SC, et al. Intramuscular nerve distribution pattern of ankle invertor muscles in human cadaver using sihler stain. *Muscle Nerve.* 2016;53(5):742—747.

Foot

32. Del Toro DR, Park TA. Abductor hallucis false motor points: electrophysiologic mapping and cadaveric dissection. *Muscle Nerve.* 1996;19(9):1138—1143.

33. Monteiro A, Cricenti SV, Manzano GM, Nobrega JA. Anatomical observations and false motor points in intrinsic foot muscles. *Muscle Nerve.* 2002;26(4):557.

34. Lee JH, Han SH, Ye JF, Lee BN, An X, Kwon SO. Effective zone of botulinum toxin a injections in hallux claw toe syndrome: an anatomical study. *Muscle Nerve.* 2012;45(2):217—221.

Index